CALISTHENICS

GREEK GOD MUSCLE BUILDING PROGRAM

BY

JOHN O'MALLEY

INTRODUCTION

I want to thank you and congratulate you for downloading the book, "Calisthenics 2.0: Greek God Muscle Building – The Ultimate Calisthenics Workout."

This book contains proven steps and strategies to gain muscle and develop incredible strength. It is by far the best calisthenics program out there. Especially if you want to maximize your strength, improve your physical capacity and build muscle. It is the result of years of research. There is no other program out there that will give you these amazing results, in a short period of time.

In this book, you will understand what calisthenics are. The main focus is on doing actual Calisthenics. This book is filled with the steps, and tips that deliver an intense program and improve your Calisthenics workout.

There is also the added information of a bank of exercises. Very specific exercises that even beginners can use. You do not need to be experience to perform the exercises. You will find just about everything you need in this book and help you set proper expectations.

If you opt to workout at a gym, looking for an instructor will be a breeze now, as you will now have an idea about the exercises you need to do.

By the end of the program, you be able to perform the hardest Calisthenics exercises, in a short period of time. I recommend you follow the program for at least 10 weeks.

Follow the principles and rules I am teaching you, and you will have the results; muscle and strength gains.

Thanks again for downloading this book, I hope you enjoy it.

TABLE OF CONTENTS

CONTENTS

Section 1:
FUNDAMENTAL PRINCIPLES AND RULES

WHAT IS CALISTHENICS?

Calisthenics is a combination of gymnastics and dance movements, to have body fitness and grace of movement. It came from the Greek word kalos meaning "beautiful," and sthenos, which means "strength." Benefits of doing Calisthenics exercises are a more intense workout that women have been doing for a long time.

When people exercise, they have the mindset to have a great figure; you must spend months at the gym or doing exercise routines daily. Calisthenics is scientifically-studied based on calorie intake and daily recommended doses of vitamins and minerals. It is a balanced result of muscle gain, in a specific time and incredible strength, with limitations of course. It also has a very positive effect on your health, as with other exercise, but with a very big difference in results.

It is a name given to repetitive exercises that use the resistance of your body to build strength; using your own strength and stretching the most out of it. It increases flexibility and burns fat. There is no equipment or weights required, and the exercises can be executed where you have space and enough floor room to move freely. Calisthenics is one of the ways to build strength and muscle mass, without using weights or heavy gym equipment. People do Calisthenics when they want to enhance or tone their body's core strength, or maintain a physically fit form; although, it is not the first choice of exercise by a body builder- they require heavy weights to build muscles.

Not to degrade body building but Calisthenics is very different from body building. If you want to be a competitive bodybuilder, including both types of training techniques will lead to the best all-around gains. The two most important factors are eating the right amount of calories and putting stress on your muscles. Calisthenics has all of this, it is simply the education of making your body healthy, fit and toned, at the same time.

Before you consider adding Calisthenics to your daily routine, here are some tips worth considering:

- When someone gets stronger, he or she has a tendency to become more flexible. In fact, you cannot become more flexible without toning and building muscle strength. A powerful muscle doesn't need to strain to contract, as a weak one must perform. Being flexible is not just twisting and flexing over things, or performing a move. It is the ability to minimize the use of strength, by using the most out of your muscle energy.

- Weight loss, one of the most talked about issues these days. Losing weight is everyone's main target in exercising. Calisthenics tackles the problem of burning excess fats from two directions. First, the strength training builds muscle mass and tones the body all over. Increased muscle mass raises your resting metabolic rate, allowing your body to burn more calories, every single moment of your exercises, every day. Second, Calisthenics causes your heart rate to rise, hence giving you more airtime control and proper breathing effect.

- One of the most beneficial effects of Calisthenics is increased endurance. Circuit training calisthenics requires you to do as many repetitions of an exercise as possible, pushing to the limit and going beyond what you can do, without rest and until one becomes fatigued. Sounds hard, right? Every day that you perform these exercises, having allowed your muscle and body to heal overnight, your endurance will increase. You will be able to perform more repetitions before fatigue is reached. When you perform evenly within all muscle groups, the result is increased endurance through every part of your body, including your cardiovascular system.

Just like any other exercise program and workouts, Calisthenics has PROS and CONS. Not everyone who works out has a goal of achieving aesthetics. For example, Calisthenics is about balance, core stability, body control and endurance of your upper and lower body. But a good Calisthenics workout also includes body weight squats and, most importantly sprinting and jumping. Sprinters don't have massive bodies or big, dense muscles, but they are performance-driven and fit for their purpose. The whole point of fitness is to find a workout regime that suits your goals and plans.

The notion that working with weights would make Calisthenics easy is not true, and it will be proved in this book. Let me ask you a question. How many strong men do you see executing 30 Pull-Ups, front lever pulls, human flags and squats? Calisthenics is a whole different skill-set to master. Let's accept that a lot of people do Calisthenics because they can't afford to enroll themselves in gym programs, or they just simply want to learn some cool bodyweight moves.

Calisthenics has goals for each individual. It can be used in many different applications; increase strength, muscular endurance, work capacity, conditioning, speed, and explosiveness. However today, Calisthenics is very under-appreciated and has almost disappeared from mainstream fitness worlds. Try asking someone what is Calisthenics; pretty sure they will end up asking you back, what it is. Then ask what Body Building is; you will get more positive answers.

Let this be your motivation to start Calisthenics as a lifestyle. Gym memberships are becoming more expensive, and it takes more of your time, and schedule. It would definitely be more expensive to buy your own equipment, and then setting it all up somewhere in your house. Compared to Calisthenics, which does not require you to purchase anything but be present and have a strong motivation.

Body weight training is safe, but you should keep in mind, that there is always a possibility of injury, if you aren't careful. Using your weight against your strength and limitations will get you to achieve your goals and satisfaction.

In Calisthenics, progress is made by moving, in order, onto more challenging movements, not by jumping onto a heavier weight. For example, starting with a Push-Up and progressing to one arm Push-Up. Incredible, right? Doing this adds a twist to exercising. It is fun and enjoyable, as well as helps build self-confidence. When you see the results of your hard work, it enhances your self-motivation, and you want to continue to see results.

It is up to you how you achieve your dream body, and live a healthy and proactive lifestyle. This book is designed to open your eyes, and demonstrate how Calisthenics can become an integral part of your life; adapt it and how to live with it. Challenge yourself to push your limits and enjoy a reward at the end. There is no such thing as perfection, all we have is righteousness. Loving and enjoying what you are doing is the key. Following a good program is different from following great tips, it is how you apply and do it.

Chapter 1:
INTENSITY — HOW HARD YOU NEED TO TRAIN

Calisthenics 2.0 is a high-intensity training plan. If you are already familiar with my work, you know that I am a "science" guy. Everything that is written and explained in this book is backed by science. I want to make sure you understand what this book is about before you continue. This book is not a 200-page book full of fluff; to make you feel smart without helping you achieve your goals. This is a results-oriented program that you need to apply. Now, if you're ready to start, you will see exactly what Calisthenics 2.0 is about. I will teach you the fundamental principles of training and everything that comes with the training. You will learn how to progress fast and do the hardest exercises. You will become more flexible, develop your core strength to do flags and levers.

The first principle I am going to teach you is; if you want to gain strength, your muscles need to be pushed to their maximum potential. If not, you won't experience massive gains. There is a point in every set where the body's ***growth mechanism*** is activated; stop before this point because NO muscular growth is stimulated after that.

Practitioners and trainers call this experience *the overload*. The necessary stimulation to force adaptation or growth occurs in the last repetition of a set. If you want to make enhance and increase muscle fibers; exert a good deal of effort! Always remember, *doing your training without going over your maximum strength level is useless.*

Let us put it this way. If you already know the maximum repetitions you can execute on a specific set is around 12, and you stopped after 8, do not expect any development. Doing anything under your maximum capability does little, to *NOTHING.* You wasted your efforts to stimulate muscle growth and strength, along with wasting your time and sweat.

If you want your body to grow bigger and stronger; train beyond your limits. This results in training with 100% intensity or what we call *muscular failure.*

"What do I mean by failure?"

Failure is the point where you cannot go on. While doing repetitions, you will reach the point where your limbs are shaking, but if you still can do it, then do it! Why? Because still being able to go on means you are merely approaching your limit, but you haven't exactly reached it yet.

In other words, failure is the moment when you can no longer execute one more rep, without assistance.

Chapter 2:
3 RULES FOR SUCCESS DURING CALISTHENICS 2.0

Volume – The Amount of Work or Sets You Will Do

You should start to understand that high-intensity stress on your muscles is fundamental to stimulating growth. You have to keep pushing yourself until you reach your limit; and that applies for every set. Thinking that you will build more muscle by doing more repetitions is not that true. It can actually hinder and can be counter-productive to muscle building. That being said, doing less than 8 repetitions is not recommended in this program.

A number of studies have concluded that 4-6 sets can result in a 40% greater hypertrophy. So, the point is: As long as you train to failure, you will stimulate growth.

Frequency – How Often to work on Each Body Part

In the first 6-week long Calisthenics 2.0 training cycle, you will do 3 sets to failure for each body part. You will train your full body this way, 3 days a week. Each body part is trained 3 times per week, with a fairly low amount of sets.

On the other days, you will do a max of 6 reps and 1 giant set, for each body part; and really blast it. You will train 4 days per week in total. You will train each body part twice per week, with a moderately high amount of sets.

The more you stimulate the muscles, the more it adapts to the growth. You push its limits and it will react by pushing back and getting stronger. Train that body part again and again, before it can retract. The main idea with training is to keep your brain two steps ahead of your body.

Staying In The Repetition Range In All Sets

Does it make sense to start your workout with easier exercises and/or less repetitions and gradually increase to harder exercises and more repetitions? No. It doesn't. It is actually counter-productive.

The only time that you have 100% of your strength intact is at the very start of your workout.

You should begin each workout with the hardest exercise and the highest number of repetitions you can complete (after your warm-up). You will achieve the highest gains when you train this way. Calisthenics 2.0 is a pyramid-style training, a REVERSE-pyramid. So how do we train?

- Warm up (3x 10 reps of easy exercises such as push-ups, jumping jacks, squats)

- Focus on a particular body part and perform the hardest exercise, with the most repetitions.

- Take a 1-2 minute break, reduce the number of repetitions and do the same exercise, or do an easier exercise with the most reps you can complete.

- For each successive set of the same exercise, you will reduce the number of repetitions.

How Do I Know When to Change Exercise Rather Than Doing Less Repetitions?

You need to stay between 8-14 repetitions for maximum muscle growth, except for certain exercises. For isometric or variations of some exercises, I will explain later, as it is a bit different.

Try to stay between 8-14 repetitions of an exercise, only change and do an easier exercise if you are unable to complete 8 repetitions.

When you return to the gym to perform this same workout again, you will notice your max strength has increased. You will notice that you have gained strength, and you can start to do harder exercises, do more repetitions.

Chapter 3:
INTRODUCTION TO THE BANK OF EXERCISES AND THE LEVEL SYSTEM

This is an important part of the program – *your bank of exercises.*

For each body part, you have different levels of exercise. Level 1 (L1) exercises are the easiest. Level 9 (L9) are the hardest.

We will use the levels differently in the 3-day routine compared to the 4-day routine, while keeping all the same principles above.

For most levels there is a variety of exercises, so you are not stuck doing the same exercises. Doing harder exercises and/ or performing more repetitions in successive workouts is the fundamental that guarantees muscle growth, fat-burning, and ultimate strength.

Beginners should start with the 3-day routine, this will help you prepare for the more advanced exercises. While the more advanced athletes should start with the 4 day routine.

Know Where You Are: Determining Your Exercise Levels

In order to start Calisthenics 2.0, you need to figure out your Level. I created this bank of exercises with different exercises for each body part, listed by Level.

Here is how you figure it out: **you are at a certain level exercise, when you can perform 14-16 reps of almost all the exercises at a Level.** I say almost, because you can have issues with performing a certain exercise when other body parts are involved.

If you already know your level, just by looking at the bank of exercises, you can begin. I recommend you do the pre-session. If you are not sure what your level is, do a pre-session before beginning a program. It will help you realize how many repetitions you can complete and give you an idea of where to start.

Pre-session 'Quickstart' guide

- If you are totally new to weight and bodyweight training, start with Level 1. Try to perform 14-16 reps of a Level 1 exercise. If you succeed, that's great! You are "L1." If it was too easy, try 14-16 reps of a Level 2 exercise. That's great! You have mastered 2 levels

- If you are new to bodyweight training, but have done weight training in the last 1 - 2 years, try to perform 14-16 reps of an L3 exercise.

- If you are not new to bodyweight training, you should know what your level is.

Section 2:
3-DAY ROUTINE

Chapter 4:
3-DAY ROUTINE

It is a total of approximately 21 sets per workout for; Monday, Wednesday, and Friday. You will do this workout for three days, every week. Rest for a full day between workouts.

I recommend you do 8 to 14 repetitions per set. You can try doing up to 16 repetitions. Once you know that you can perform 14 repetitions, without feeling strained, add a couple more repetitions. This method is better than pushing yourself to perform a hard exercise and do 2 repetitions for every 3 sets.

- Make sure you record: the number of repetitions, the exercise, and level. This is to avoid losing track of your limitations and capabilities.

- Take a 2 minute rest between every set

- It is a must that you train each body part in the exact same order.

- You will work each body part with 3 sets

Here is the important part:

For the first set, you will do an exercise that is harder than the exercise **you will do for the last 2 repetitions**.

For example, if you just start and have 3 sets for Chest, you will do a Level 2 (L2) exercise like Push-Ups for the first set, then do 2 sets of an L1 exercise, such as Inclined Push-Ups.

At the beginning, learn how to perform each new exercise. Take the time to learn. Practice, fail, and do it again until you succeed.

The Rule

If you can perform 16 repetitions without going to failure at your first set, go to the next level.

Example: Chest: Day 1:

Level 2 (L2) exercise x1 set (Push-Ups) / L1 exercise x2 sets (Inclined Push-Ups).

If you do 16 repetitions of the L2 exercise (Push-Ups), next time you train your chest, you will do: Level 3 (L3) exercise x1 set (such as Declined Push-Ups) /L2 exercise x2 sets (Push-Ups).

Calisthenics 2.0: 3-Day Workout

Order of the body parts you will train in this 3-day workout regime:

- Legs
- Chest
- Abs
- Obliques
- Back and shoulders

NOTE: There are no isolated shoulders exercises, as they are involved in almost all exercises; especially the back, the chest, and triceps.

- Biceps

- Triceps

Beginners: you will perform Level 2 (L2) exercises for each body part for the first set, then perform Level 1 (L1) exercises for each body part for the last 2 sets.

3-Day Routine Example

If you have completed the pre-session and figured out your level.

Legs: Level 5

Chest: Level 4

Abs: Level 4

Obliques: Level 3

Back and shoulders: Level 3

Biceps: Level 3

Triceps: Level 4

This could be your workout for Monday, Wednesday and Friday:

NOTE: 8-12 reps- always until failure

- Pistols

- Single Leg Burpee

- Single Leg Burpee

- Wide-grip crucifix Push-Up

- Spiderman Push-Up

- Spiderman Push-Up

- Marcus Bondi Ab crunches
- V-up
- V-up

- Side oblique crunches
- Spiderman Push-Up
- Spiderman Push-Up

- Sternum Pull-Up
- Side to side Pull-Up
- Side to side Pull-Up

- Negative Chin-Up
- Body biceps curl
- Body biceps curl

- Diamond Push-Up
- Triceps bar-extension
- Triceps bar extension

Section 3:
THE 4-DAY WORKOUT

Chapter 5:
THE CALISTHENICS 2.0, 4-DAY ROUTINE

- Monday: Chest/Back & Shoulders
- Wednesday: Legs/Arms/Abs
- Friday: Chest/Back & Shoulders
- Sunday: Legs/Abs /Obliques

Stick to this order, it's well-designed for increasing strength and muscle growth, while burning fat. This regime focuses on working your abs; make them firm and stronger.

You will work on each body part twice per week, with a maximum of 7 sets, except for arms. There will be an arms session Wednesday; as we want to work on them properly, at least once a week, to their maximum potential.

Continue to work between 8-14 repetitions. More if necessary, not less, except when you are learning to execute a new exercise (especially for those who have just started bodyweight training).

Continue to keep track of: number of repetitions, exercises you perform, and level.

The Way You will Work for The First 6 Sets

Here is what you will do for the first 6 sets. Do you remember the reverse-pyramid style? This principle is very important in the 4-day program.

Let me explain further. **For each body part:**

- **Do the REVERSE-PYRAMID LEVEL** for the **first** *three* **sets**

- **Do it twice**

What does that mean?

Example: **Chest day:** Perform Level 3 exercises for your first set, followed by Level 2 exercises for your second set, then Level 1 exercises for your third set.

How do I determine the level of exercises I to start with?

You need to stay between 8-14 repetitions. If you are able to complete 20-22 repetitions of **Level 2 (L2)** exercise, 12-14 repetitions of **Level 3 (L3)** exercise, but only 5-7 repetition of **Level 4 (L4)** exercise, you will start with L3 exercise.

That is the plan for the first 3 sets. You will complete this round of 3 sets twice. Then decrease the level for the next round.

Example: At your best, you can perform 12-14 repetitions of a L4 exercise for chest, such as one-arm Push-Ups.

You can do the following (to your limit):

- 1x One-arm Push-Up (L4 exercise)

- 1x Muscle-Up (L3 exercise)

- 1x Deep Dip (L2 exercise)

- 1x Muscle-Up (L3 exercise)

- 1x Deep Dip (L2 exercise)

- 1x Push-Up (L1 exercise)

Note: If you are unable to complete 8-14 repetitions of the L4 exercise, perform the following:

- 1x L3

- 1x L2

- 1x L1

- 1x L2

- 1x L1

- 1x L1

Take a 3 minute rest between rounds; perform the second round with more strength.

What You Will Do for The Last Set

That's it for the first 6 sets. For the last set, you won't do a regular set but a superset or what we call a '*giant set.*'

If you can perform, at your best, 12-14 repetitions of L4 exercise, you can now do a superset of L4-L3, or a giant set of L3-L2-L1. Feel free to change them, depending on the needs of your body. This will ensure your muscle has no choice but to grow as you push yourself to the limit and go to failure. Also, do not forget to **push hard**.

That's it for the 4-day routine. Now let's go to the bank of exercises.

Section 4:
BANK OF EXERCISES

Bank of exercises, as we know, sometimes depends on your strengths and weaknesses. Still I decided to create this bank of exercises listed by levels and I'm confident enough to say that if you don't have a real weakness, this bank of exercises could not be more accurate.

Biceps

Level 1 Exercise (For Beginners)

Isometric Body Bicep Curl (with Rings or Straight Bar, Feet on The Ground)

First, your feet should be spread apart, and lined up under your hips. Hold the resistance bands, with your palms facing forward, position your arms freely at your sides. Stand tall, tuck your tummy in and bend your knees a bit. Flex both of your arms upward until your hands are level with your shoulders and maintain that position. Once you complete a rotation, return to your original position. Focus on the elbow flexion- the more vertical that you do it, the easier it is for you.

Rings:

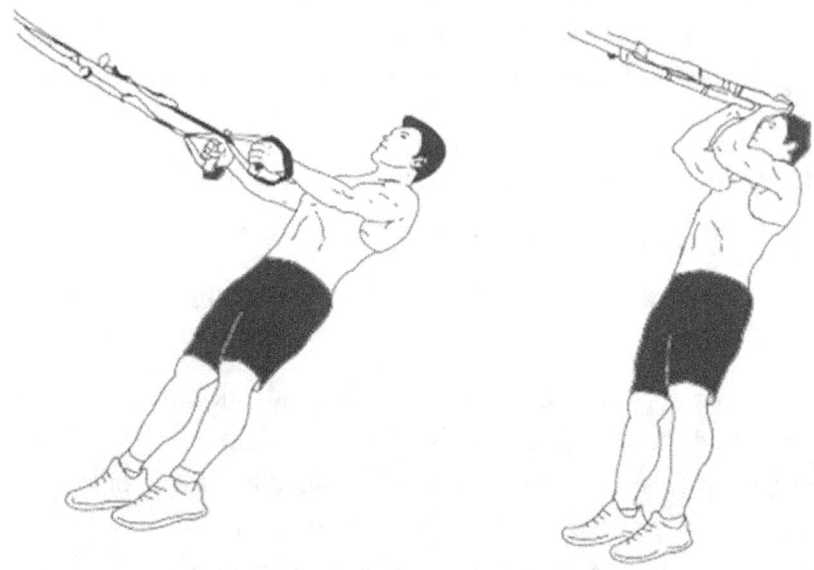

Straight bar:

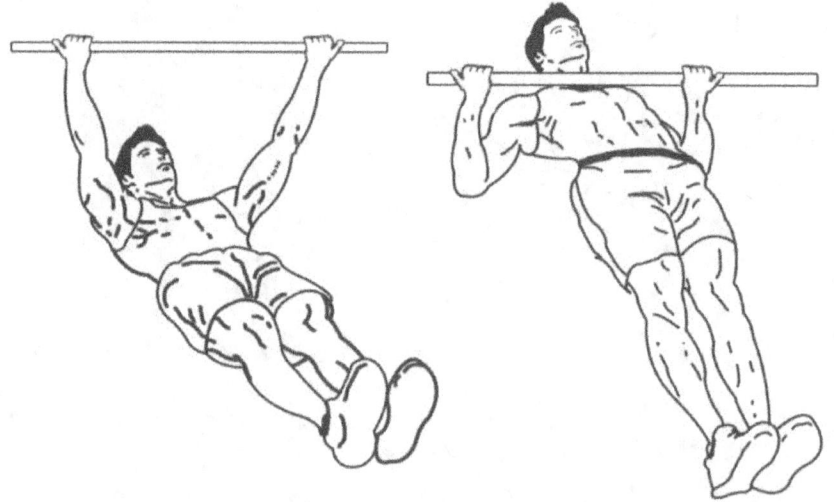

Level 2 Exercise

Isometric Chin-Up (1 sec = 1 rep)

You will need a horizontal bar or chin-up bar, positioned above your shoulder height. Grip the bar, palms face your body. Lift your body using your arm strength, until your chin passes the bar. Your knees should be bent, for weight distribution. Keep the same position for 15 seconds or more. Lower yourself back to the ground.

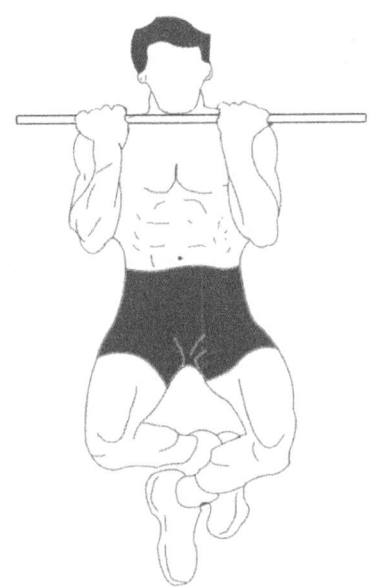

Level 3 Exercise

Body Bicep Curls (Straight Bar/Rings, Feet on the Ground)

Your feet should be apart and lined up under your hips. Hold the resistance bands, with your palms facing forward, position your arms freely at your sides. Stand tall, tuck your tummy in and knees bent a bit. Flex both of your arms upward until your hands are level with your shoulders, then return to your original position. Focus on the elbow flexion because the more vertical that you do it, the easier it is for you.

Rings:

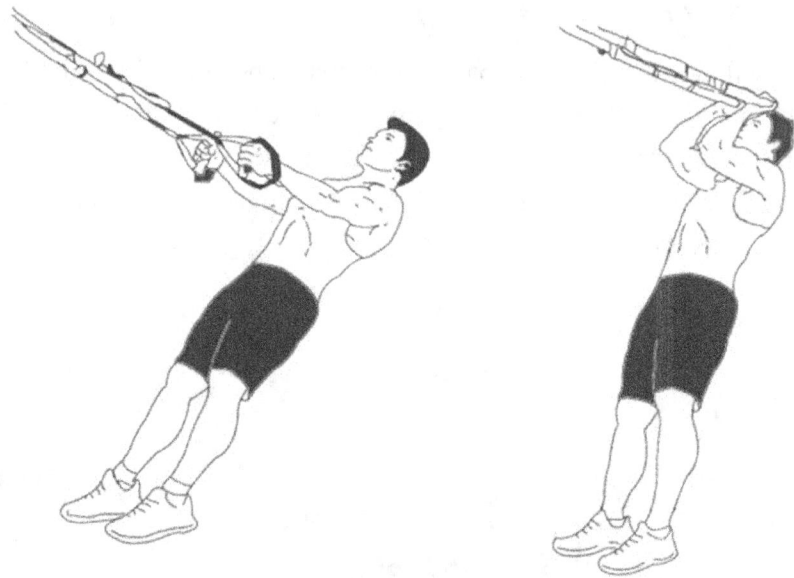

Straight bar:

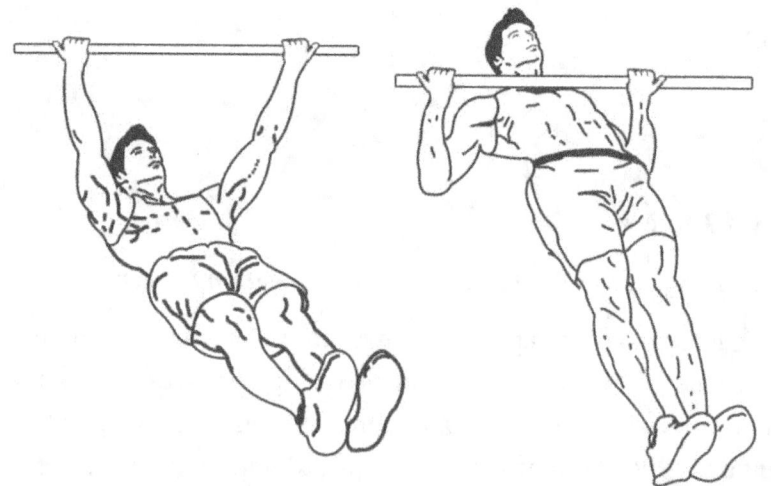

Level 4 Exercises

Negative Chin-Up (Supinated-Grip Pull-Up) (For this exercise, 1 negative rep = 7 reps)

You will need a horizontal bar for this. Pull yourself up to the bar, hands facing you. Do this as far as you can from the bar. Make sure your collarbone is above the bar, then lower yourself back to the ground, as slow as you can (around 8 seconds).

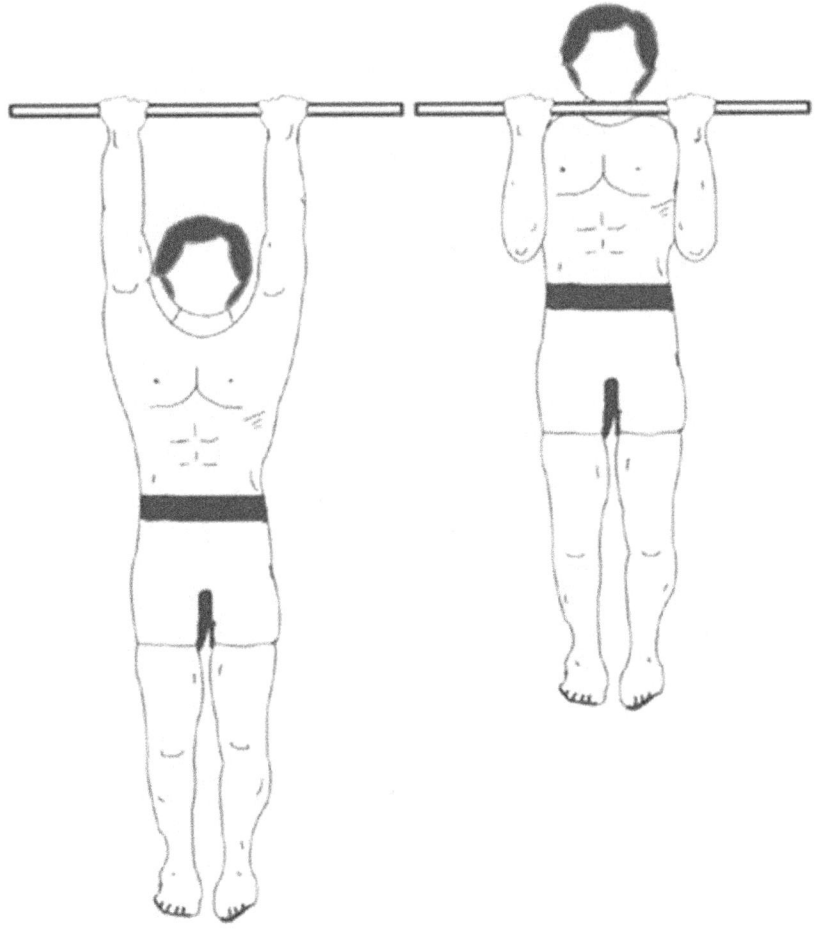

Negative Closed Grip Chin-Up

Same exercise as above, with a closed-grip.

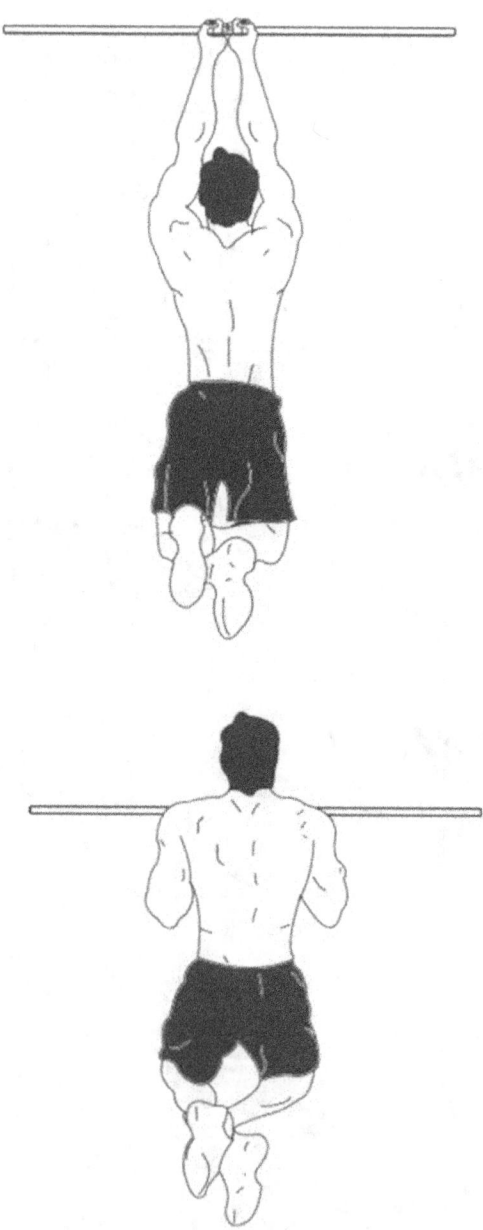

Level 5 Exercises

Chin-Up (Supinated-Grip Pull-Up)

You will need a horizontal bar for this. Pull yourself up to the bar, hands facing you. Do this as far as you can from the bar. Make sure your collarbone is above the bar and then lower yourself back to the ground.

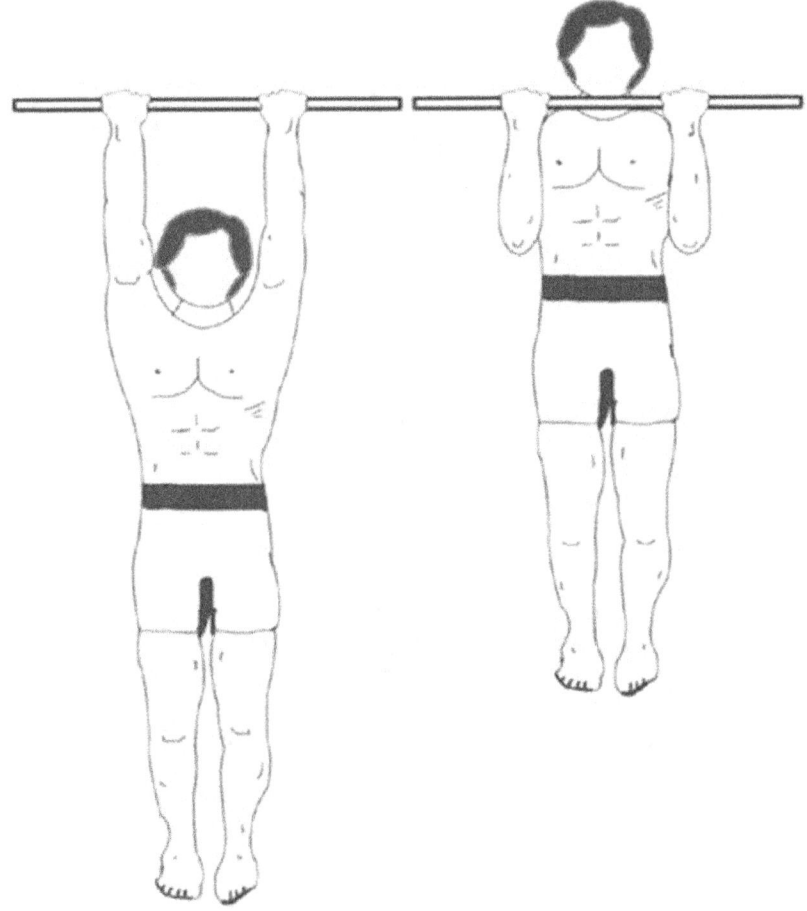

Closed Grip Chin-Up

Grip the pull-up bar with arms facing you and pull your whole body weight up until your chin is above the bar. Lower yourself, make sure that your arms are fully extended.

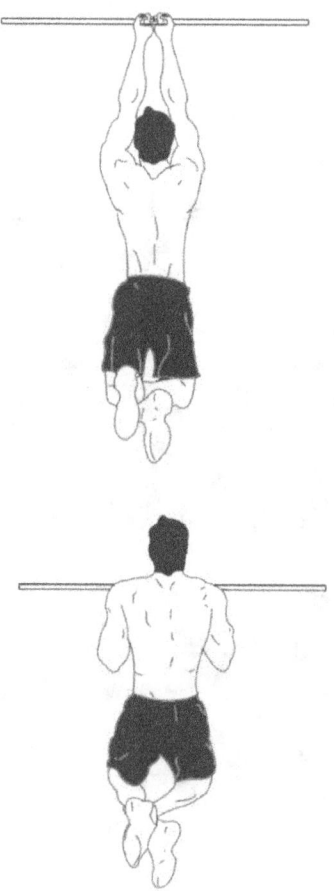

Level 6 Exercise

Tucked Front Lever Pull

Like any other static hold, the Tuck Front Lever Pull activates many muscle groups at once. Learning, understanding and maintaining a good form is very important in bodyweight training. There are two main strengths needed when doing the Tuck Front Lever Pull: vertical pulling strength and horizontal pulling strength. The vertical pulling strength is required for efficient climb-ups and muscle-ups, which are the two most important skills in your training. Horizontal pulling strength is also important because it comes with different skills, such as leg-ups, underbars and pull-overs. It is also needed for any movement while suspended under a bar. This is a golden exercise. I will spend enough time explaining the movement and the progression.

Tuck Front Lever Pull is the starting point for advancing to the Fully Extended Front Lever.

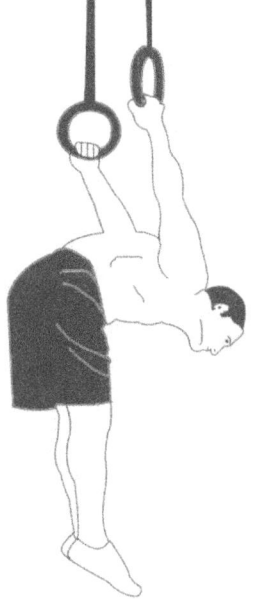

Steps to Follow:

Step 1: Grasp a high bar, with an overhand hold and suspend yourself, focus up to the sky or ceiling; make sure your tongue remains pressed against your upper pallet and jaw closed (this will help to keep the neck in position).

Step 2: While leaning back, use your biceps, back muscles and lats to pull your hips and legs up to the bar, then lower back down. Make sure your knees are tucked into your chest, and your head and chest are dropped backward to line your torso parallel with the ground. Keep the position for a few seconds then return to the starting position.

Headbanger

Hold the horizontal bar, with both hands facing away from you and pull yourself up until your chin passes the bar. Do not go back down, instead hold this height and extend your upper back and head away from the bar, as far as you can. Now, pull yourself as close as you can to the bar.

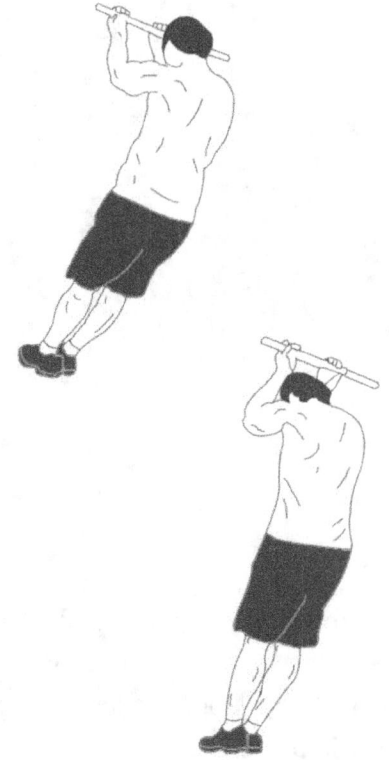

Level 7 Exercises

One-Arm Pull-Up (Assisted)

Grip the bar using your dominant hand, palms facing you. Contract your abs and pull yourself up until your chin passes the bar. Lower your body back down. Your other hand will give you extra support. Switch arms and repeat the steps above.

Side to Side Chin-Up

Grab the horizontal bar, palms facing you, and your hands wider than shoulder width. The movement is the exact same as the one-arm Pull-Up (assisted). Contract your abs, pull your body up and over the bar, to the left, until your chin passes the bar then immediately to the right. Repeat without touching the ground.

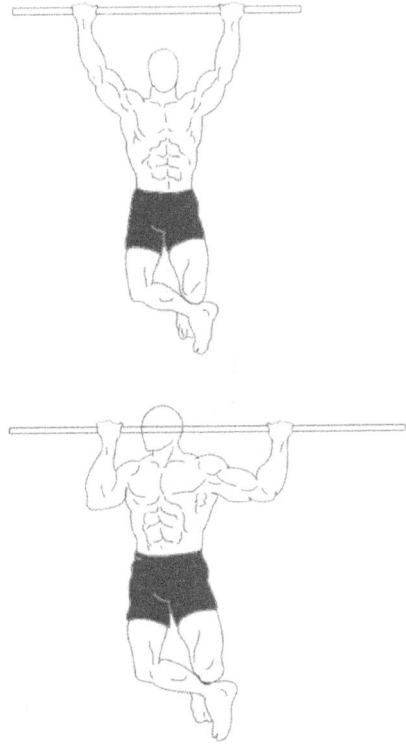

Level 8 Exercise

One-Legged Front Lever Pull

Steps to Follow:

Step 1: Grasp a high bar with an overhand hold and suspend yourself, as you focus to the sky or ceiling; make sure your tongue remains pressed against your upper pallet and jaw closed (this will help to keep the neck in position).

Step 2: Completely extend and straighten out one leg. The extended leg, back and hips should be in a straight line and parallel to the ground. Put the foot of the other leg on the knee extended leg, to form an acute angle.

Step 3: While leaning back, use your biceps, back muscles and lats to pull your hips and legs up to the bar. Make sure the bent leg is tucked in hard to your chest while the other leg remains straight and suspended in the air. Keep the position for a few seconds then return to the starting position. Switch legs and repeat the above steps.

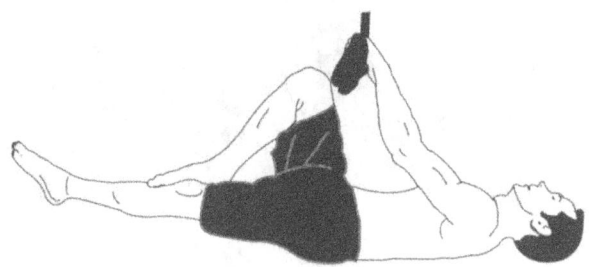

Level 9 Exercise

Front Lever Pull

Steps to Follow:

Step 1: Begin the workout at the highest point of a Pull-Up, placing your chin over the bar; arms completely bent with your body hanging and the legs extended.

Step 2: From this position, endeavor to push your shoulders as far back behind your hands, then lift your hips to a horizontal position. As the body elevates in the front, the head should remain neutral and your back should be flat, without any pikes in the hips. The elbows should locked at the horizontal position.

Step 3: Return your chin over the bar by lowering your hips and pulling back down with your arms. Make a point to finish every rep by bringing your feet back under your body.

Step 4: Pull yourself up with your arms so your midsection/chest area is as close to the bar as you can get. Gradually lower your arms down.

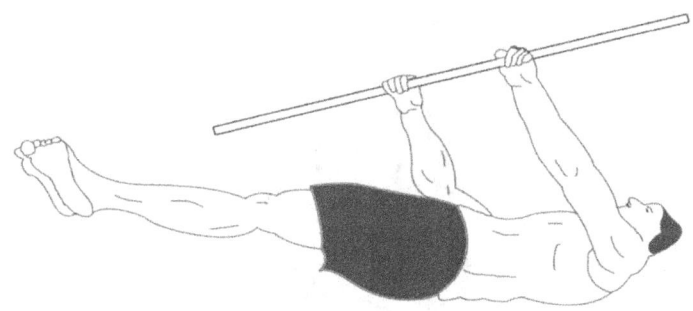

Additional Information

- Do not permit your feet to stay forward when your jaw is over the bar. For individuals looking to develop this exercise, it adds an intensity when you snap your feet gradually behind you, toward the end of every rep.

- Ensure that you rest between sets and particularly after the jaw over-the-bar position.

This exercise is really great for biceps, but requires a lot of core. If you don't have enough strength, focus on side to side chin-ups.

Level 10 Exercise

One-Arm Pull-Up/One-Arm Chin-Up (#1 Favorite Exercise To Build Your Biceps)

Grip the Pull-Up bar with one hand, then place your free hand against your back. Pull up, stay 1 second then go back down.

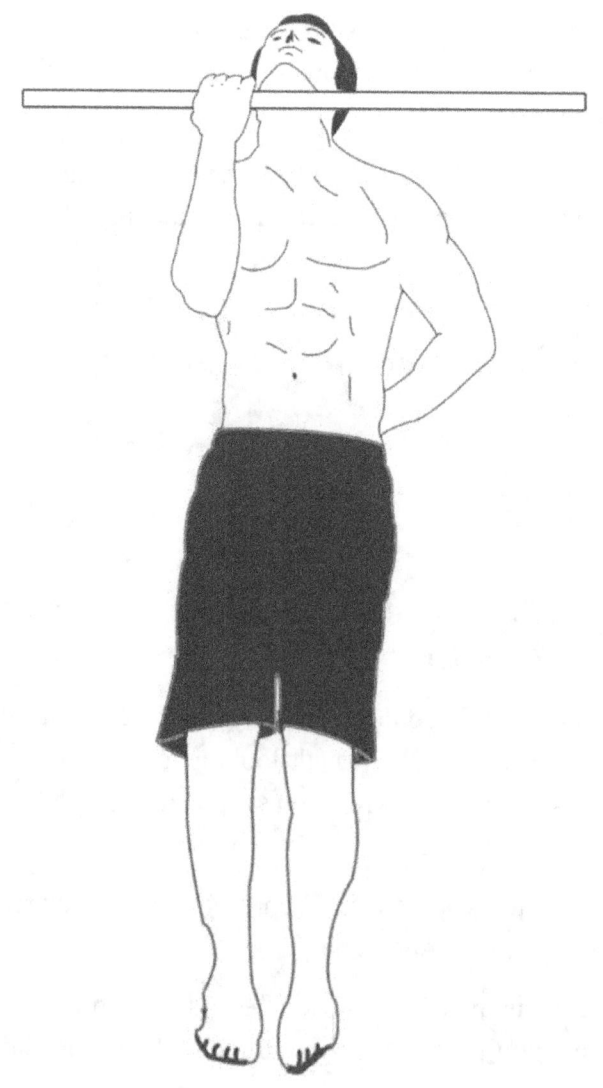

Chest

Level 1 Exercises

Inclined Push-Up

Stand in front of a bench or platform. Place your hands at the edge, a bit wider than shoulder width. Push your forefoot away from the bench/platform, until your body is fully extended. Lower your body down, bending your elbows, until your chest is almost touching the bench or platform, then return to your starting position. Make sure that when you push back up, your arms are fully extended.

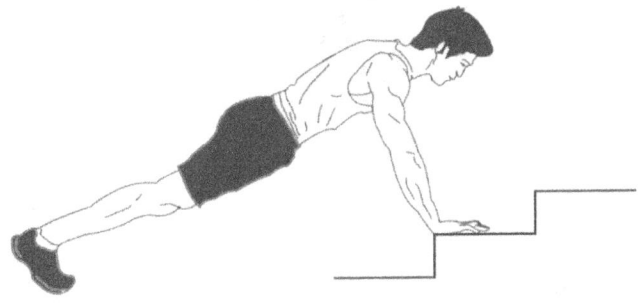

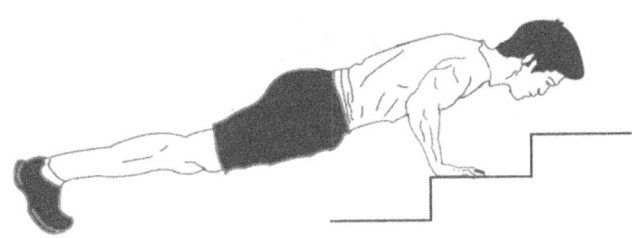

Push-Up on the Knees

Assume the regular Push-Up position, and bend your knees until they touch the ground. (You can cross your ankles to add extra intensity.) Make sure your back is straight. Bending your elbows, lower your body to the ground, and hold for 2 seconds, then return to your starting position. Make sure that when you push back up, your arms are fully extended.

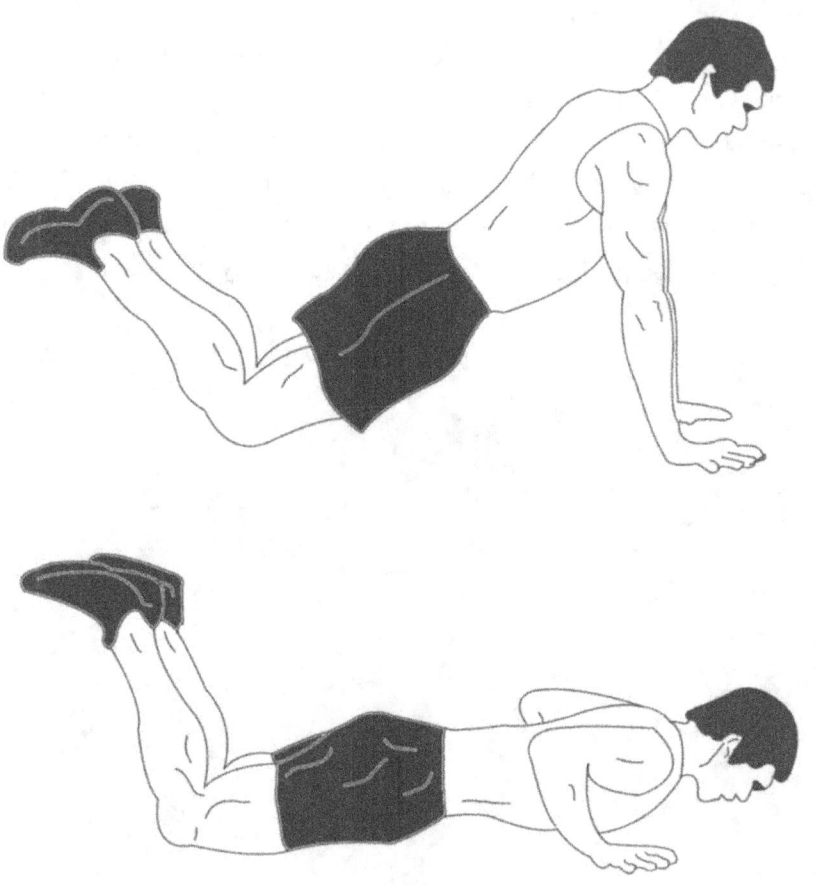

Level 2 Exercise

Push-Up

Lay your body on the ground, in a prone position, both hands flat on the ground spread a bit wider than shoulder width. Push up to fully extend your arms. Keep your back straight while lowering to the ground as you bend at the elbows. Return to starting position, arms fully extended.

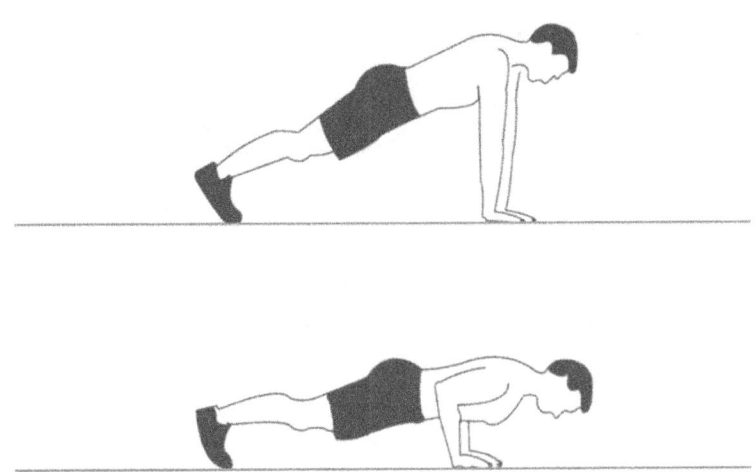

Level 3 Exercise

Explosive Clap Push-Up

Place your body in a Push-Up position, with your hands a bit wider than shoulder width. Lower your body, by bending your elbows, until your chest is about to touch the ground. Push yourself up quickly, your hands will briefly leave the ground, and clap. Return to the ground with your arms extended.

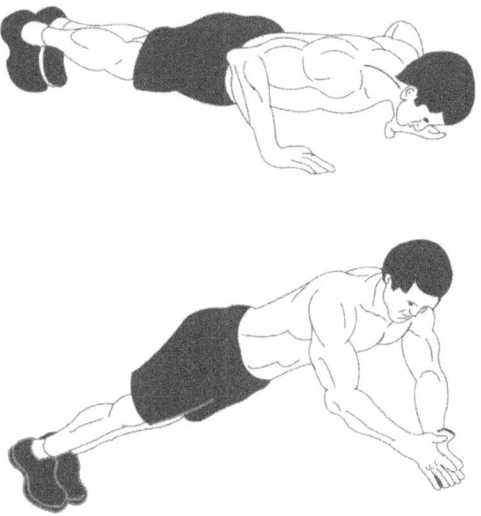

Level 4 Exercise

Wide-Grip Shoulder-Tap Push-Up

Place your body in a wide-grip Push-Up position, with your hands a bit wider than shoulder width. Lower your body to the ground, until your chest almost touches the ground. Push your upper body up until arms are fully extended, then quickly tap your opposite shoulder. Quickly return your hand to the ground. You can also do a regular Shoulder-Tap Push-Up to start, that involves the triceps more.

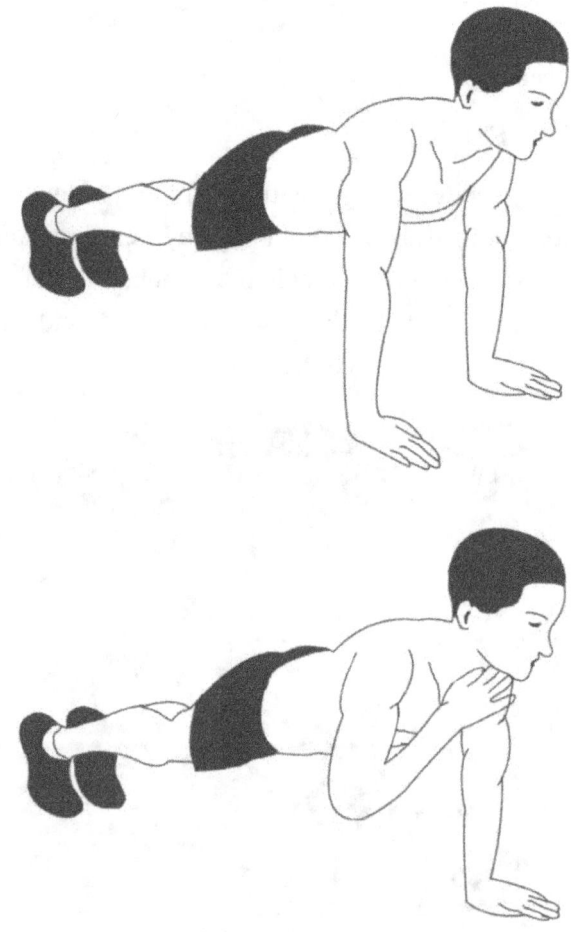

Level 5 Exercise

Spiderman Push-Up

Place your body in a Push-Up position, with your hands a bit wider than shoulder width. As you lower your body, bend your elbows, at the same time, lift your right foot off the floor, bend your knee and line your knee up to your elbow- the inside of your leg should face the ground. Return your leg to start position and lower your body down to the ground. This exercise isn't really harder than the previous one, but it's good to master it.

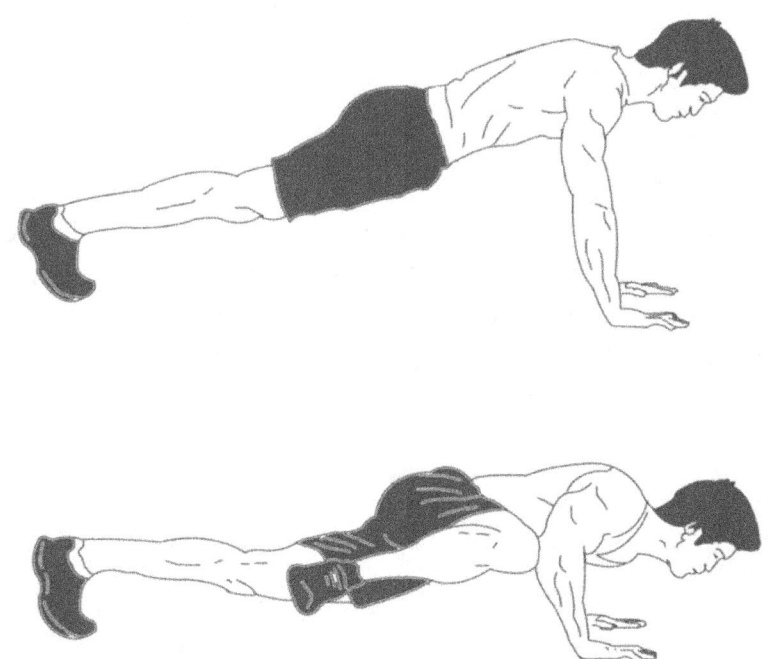

Level 6 Exercise

Wide Grip/Crucifix Push-Up (the wider, the harder)

Lie on your stomach and place your arms at your side- perpendicular to your torso. Perform a Push-Up using your fingertips and thumbs.

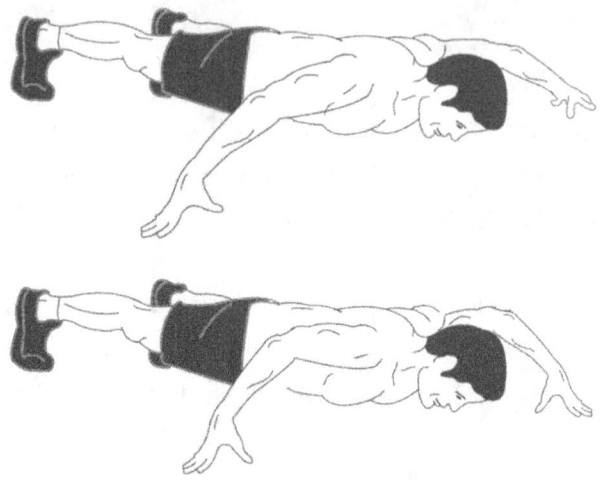

Level 7 Exercise

Deep Dip

You need two parallel, fixed and stable dip bars. Avoid doing Deep Dips between benches or on rings- can injure your shoulders. Use parallel bars that are firm and stable. Apart from the chest, Deep Dip also works your shoulders and back. If you want to avoid chest and shoulder pain then proper Deep Dip is the answer. Deep Dips will enable you to gain overall strength and muscle.

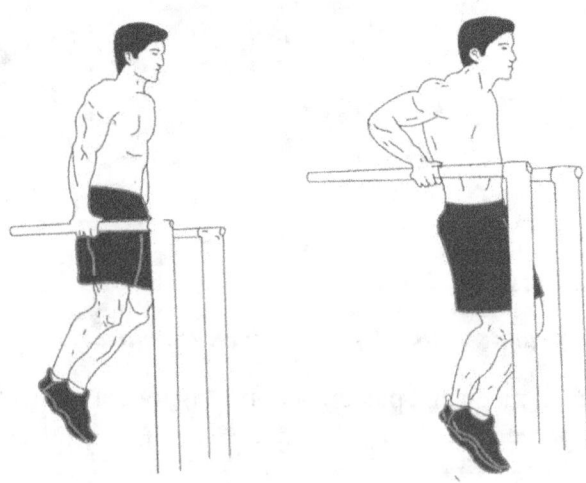

Steps to Follow:

Step 1: Grab the two parallel bars and jump up to starting position; make sure your arms/elbows are locked and straight, this will help to balance your body.

Step 2: While inhaling, lower your body slowly as you bend your arms and lean into a 30-degree angle. Go down until shoulders are below your elbows or until you feel a slight stretch in your chest.

Step 3: While exhaling, use your chest to push yourself up to the starting position, straightening your arms.

Step 4: With your shoulders above your hands, balance yourself with arms/elbows locked.

<u>*N/B:*</u> Remember to press the chest for one second while at the top of the movement.

Muscle-Up

Hold the bar by using a false grip. (False grip is your thumb on top of the bar, not around it.) Pull your body up and roll over onto the bar, then press your hands down while you are driving your body up to make a dip.

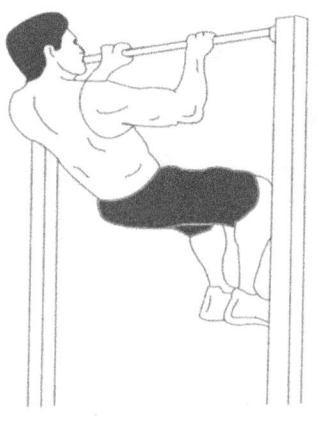
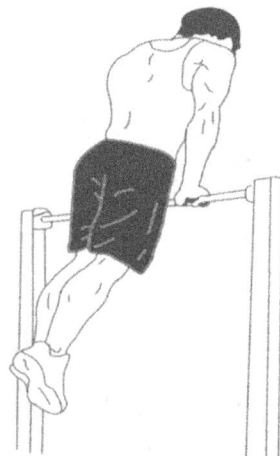

Level 8 Exercises

One-Arm Push-Up

Place your body in normal Push-Up position on the floor, place one hand against your lower back. Start with your feet apart wider than shoulder width. This makes it easier. Once you begin to gain the strength, move your feet closer, and closer together. Do a Push-Up. (When starting, a trick to make it easier- grab your bottom instead of your lower back.)

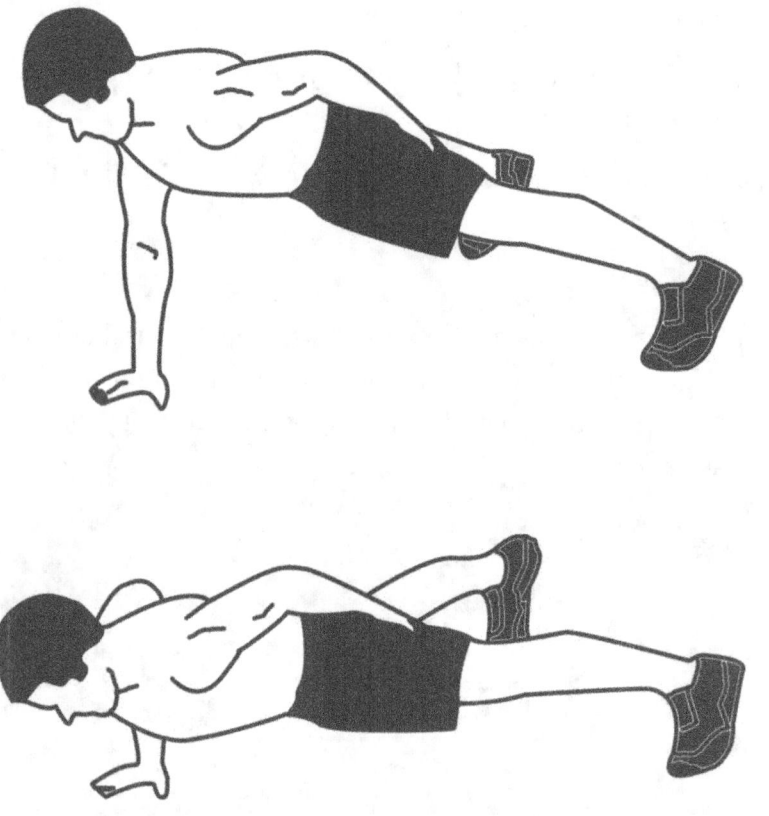

Inclined, One-Arm Push-Up

Place your body in a normal Push-Up position against a bench or platform, drape one arm across your lower back. Start with your feet a bit wider than shoulder width. This makes it easier. Perform a Push-Up. (As you become stronger with the position, move your feet closer together.)

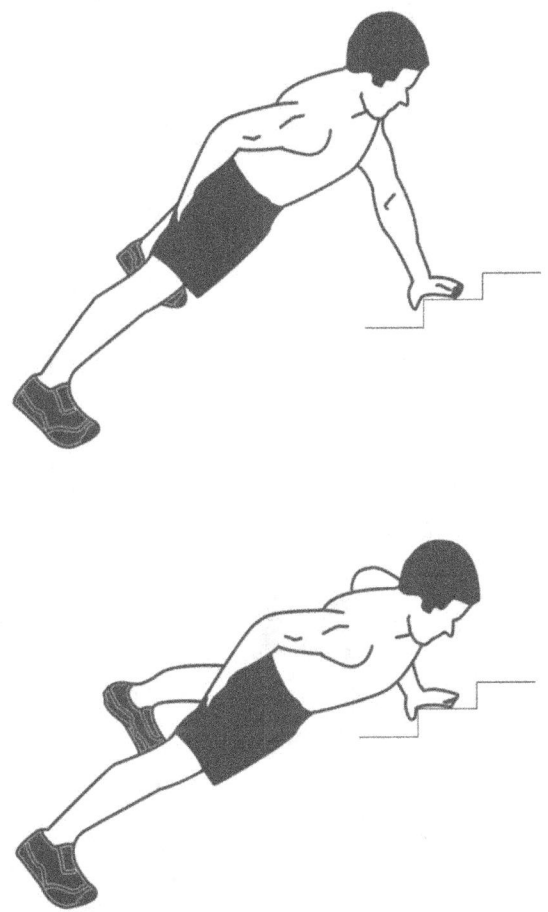

Negative Muscle-Up (1 negative=2 regular reps)

Hold the bar by using a false grip. (False grip is your thumb on top of the bar, not around it.) Pull your body up and roll over onto the bar, then press your hands down while you are driving your body up to make a dip. Lower your chest to the bar and go back to the initial position, as slow as possible.

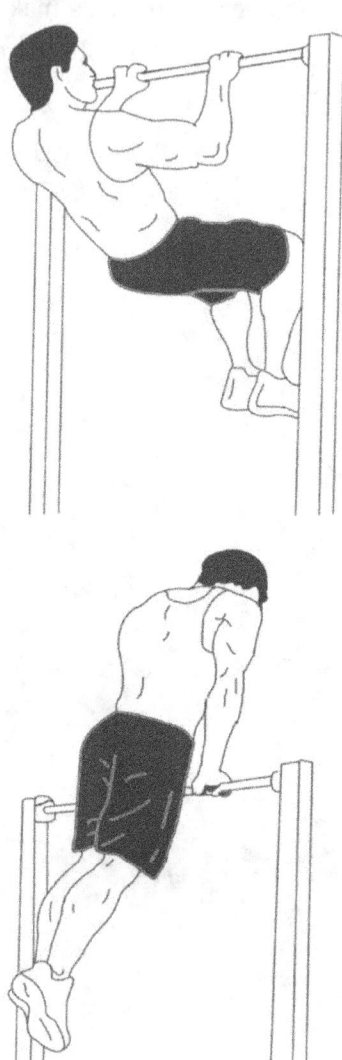

Level 9 Exercises

Negative Muscle-Up (1 negative=1 regular rep)

Hold the bar by using a false grip. (False grip is your thumb on top of the bar, not around it.) Pull your body up and roll over onto the bar, then press your hands down while you are driving your body up to make a dip. Lower your chest to the bar and go back to the initial position, as slow as possible.

One-Arm Push-Up (Feet as wide as your shoulder width)

Place your body in normal Push-Up position on the floor, drape one arm across your lower back. Perform a Push Up.

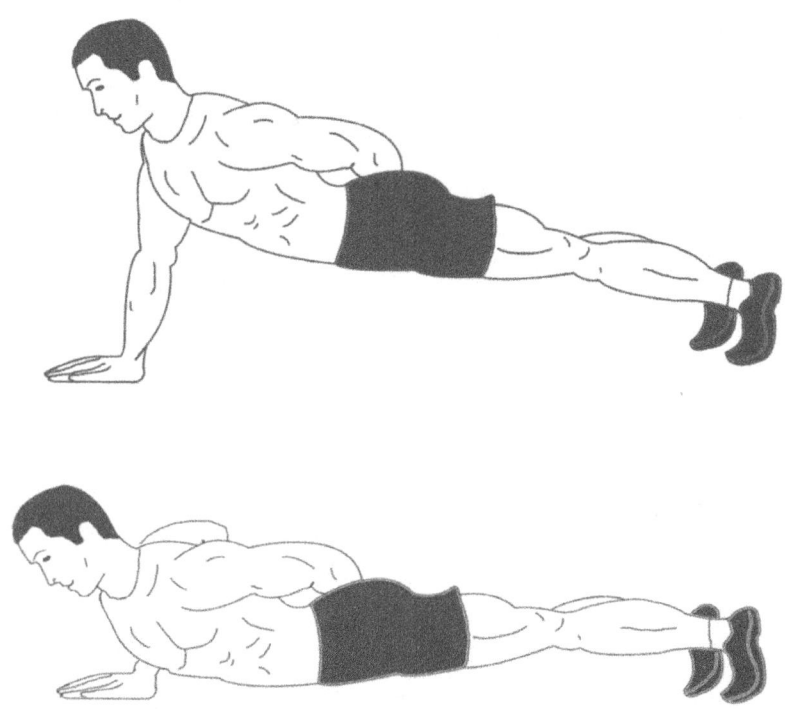

Level 10 Exercise

At this level:

Use varying angles, volumes, and tempo of the previous levels.

Do some variations of the previous exercise or create your own variations.

My advice: use chains, add weight.

ABS

Level 1 Exercise

Inclined Crunches

You are going to need a bench, in an inclined position. Lay back on the bench, bend both your legs and rest your feet against the wall, feet even with your hips. Cross your arms over your chest. Slowly raise your chest, shoulders and head off the bend, at the same time. Do not bend your lower back. Hold your position at the top of the crunch, for 2 – 4 seconds. Repeat crunches without letting your back touch the bench.

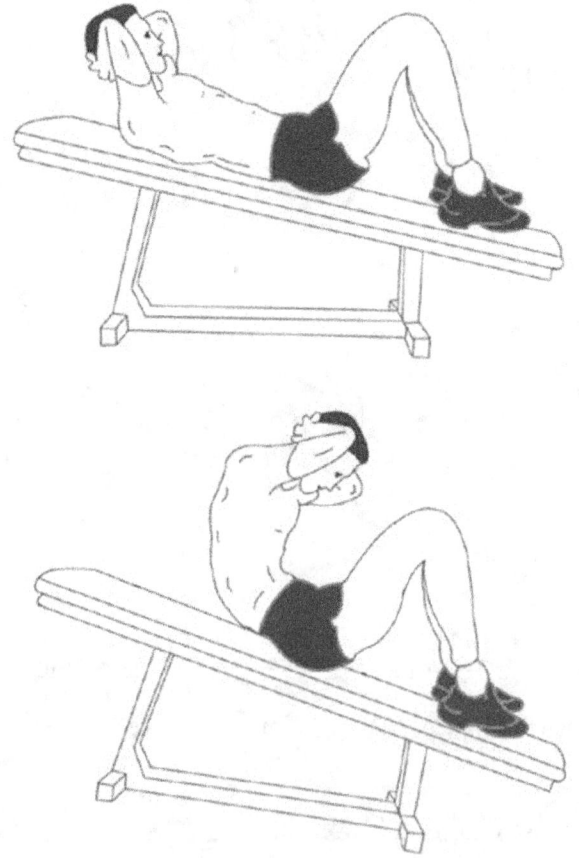

Level 2 Exercises

Crunches

Lie on the floor, feet flat on the floor, knees bent. Hands placed at the back of your head and your thumbs behind your ears. Elbows should be at your sides, but rounded in a bit. Slightly tilt your chin and pull your tummy in. Curl yourself up and raise your upper body forward. Hold this position for 2-4 seconds. Repeat crunches without letting your back touch the ground.

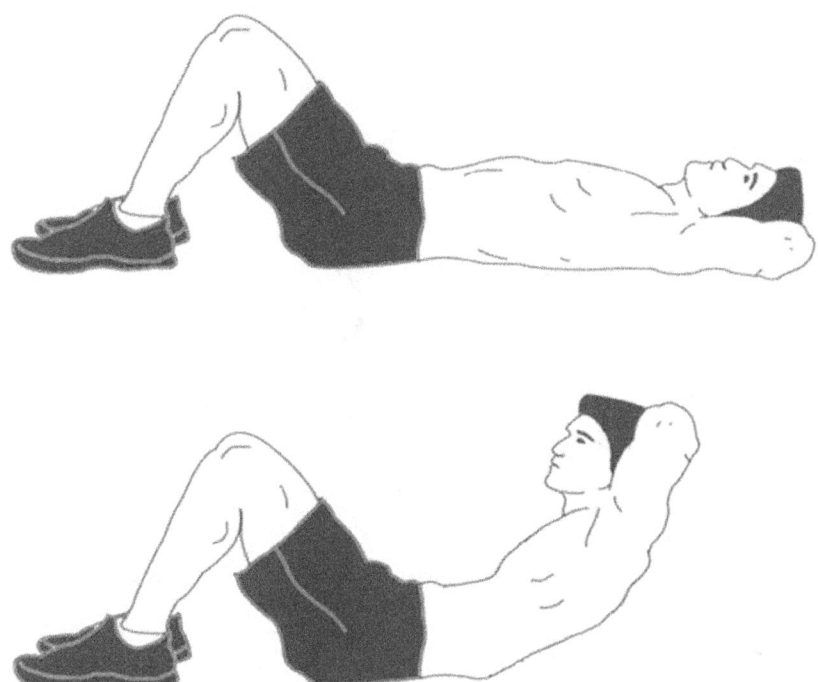

Leg Raises

Lie on your back on the floor, with your hands flat on the floor and at your sides. Bend your knees, raise your leg while contracting your abdominal muscles. Straighten your legs pointing up and slowly lower them. Repeat leg raises without letting your feet touch the ground.

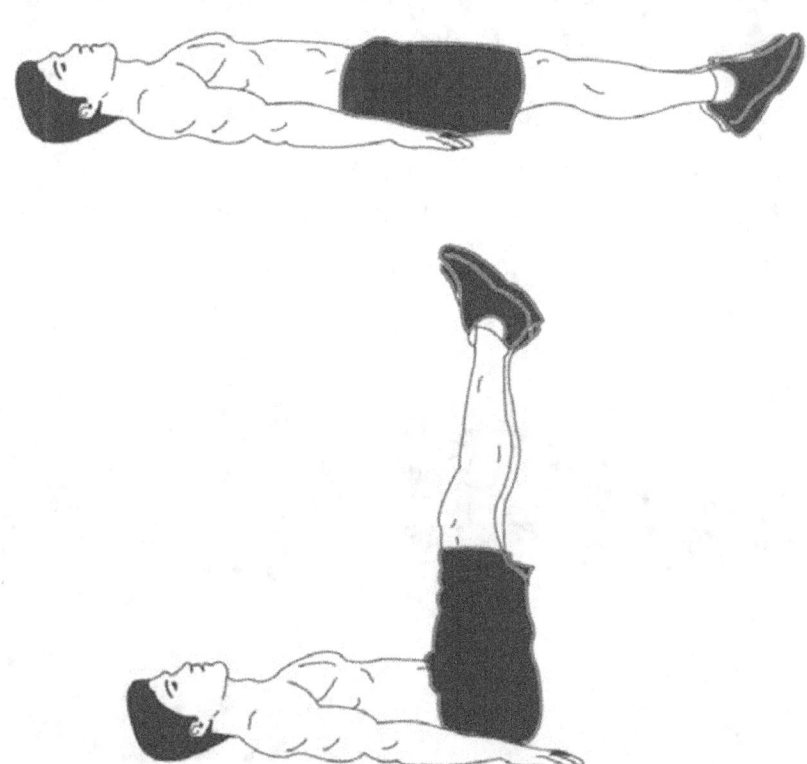

Level 3 Exercise

Declined Crunches

Lay your back against a decline bench. Secure your legs and place your hands on each side of your head. Keep your elbows in and push the small of your back down onto the bench. Pull in your abdominal muscles, as tight as you can and roll your shoulders up and off the decline bench. Exhale while doing this and keep your lower back on the decline bench. Hold the contraction for 2-4 seconds and lower yourself back to the starting point.

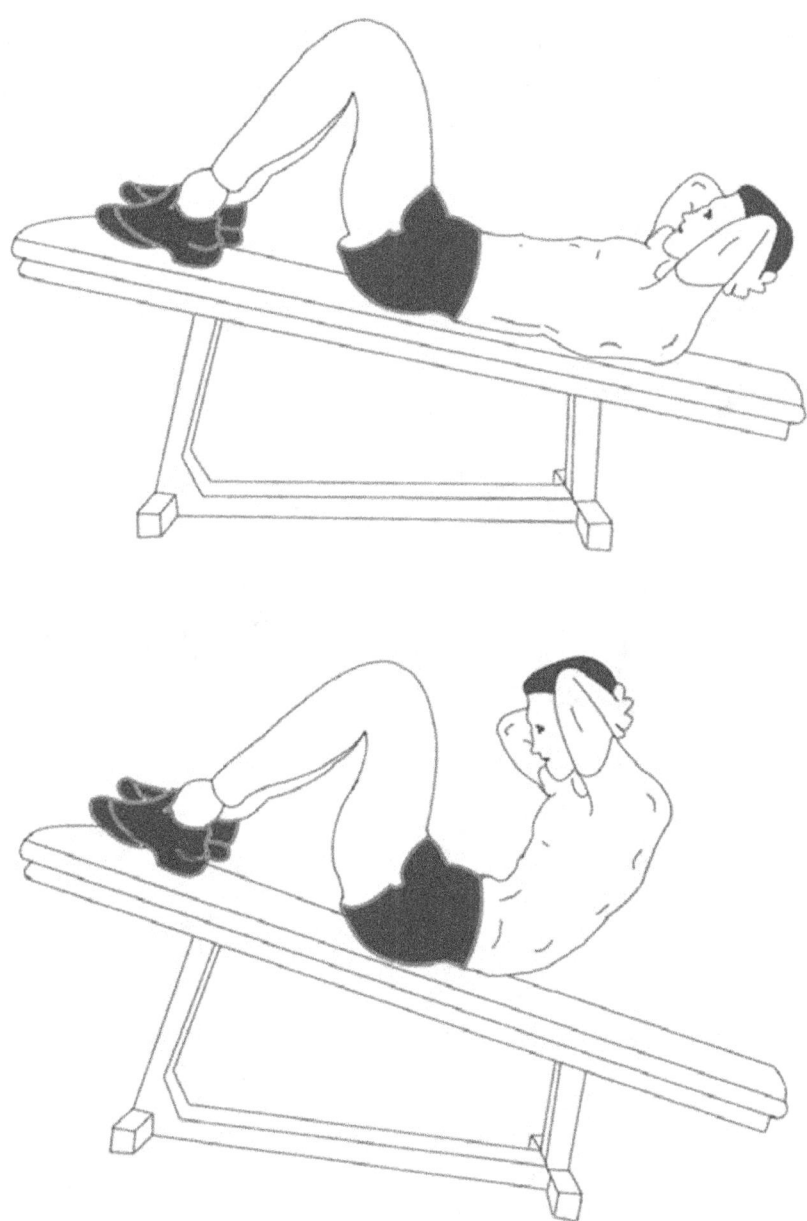

Level 4 Exercises

Knees Raises

Grab the bar with your arms fully extended. Raise your knees up and make sure not to swing your hips forward. Then return to your starting position.

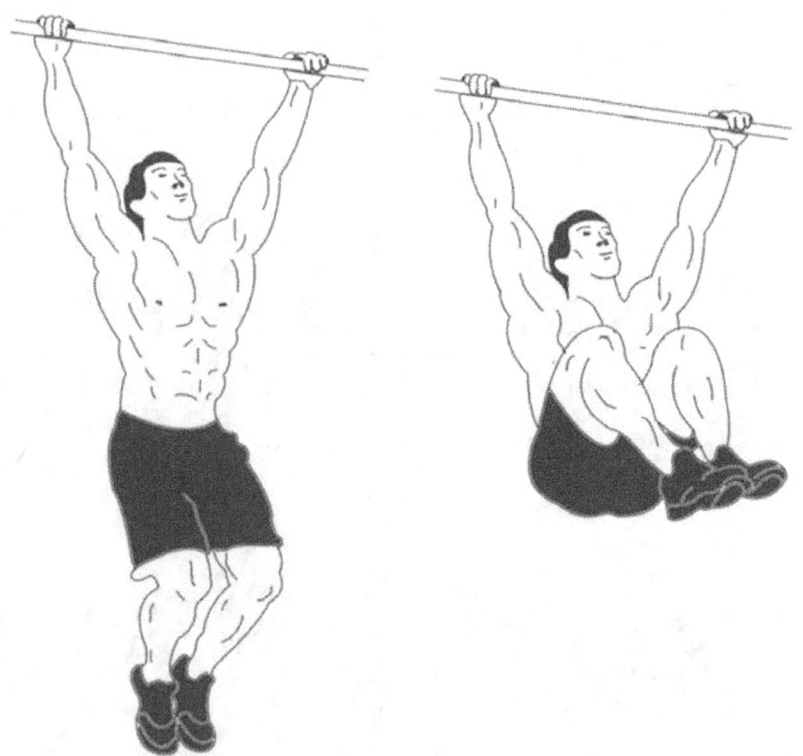

Level 5 Exercise

V-Ups

Lie on the floor with your back flat, extend your hands straight up beside your head. Extend your legs and EXHALE, while bending your waist. Raise your arms and legs and hold this position for 1 second. Lower your arms and legs back down, while INHALING.

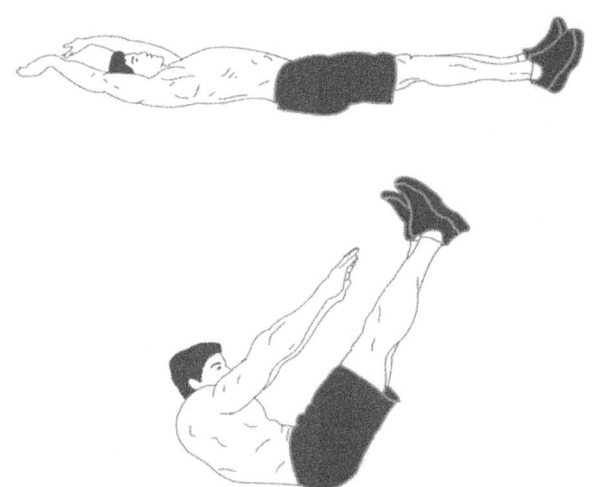

Level 6 Exercise

Marcus Bondi Ab Crunches

Going to use parallel bars to perform this exercise. Lean your upper arm against the bar, grab a bar in each hand. Raise your legs until you are in L-position, thrust your knees away from your body and then back to your chest.

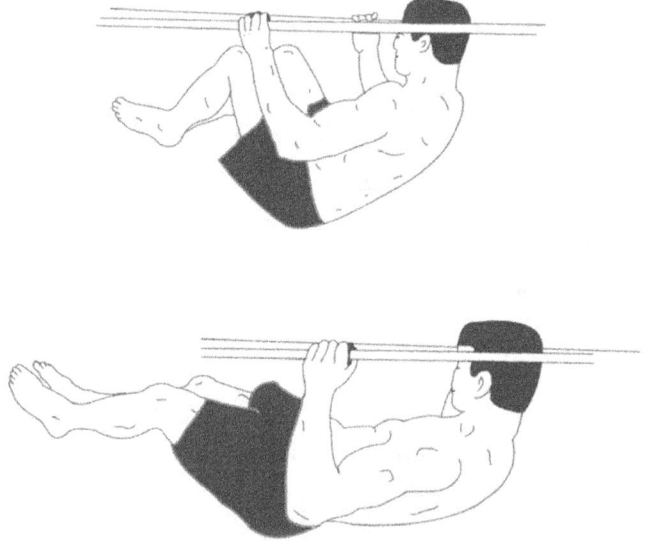

L-Sit Lifts

Grab the bar with your arms fully extended. Raise your legs until your body forms an "L". Go back and repeat.

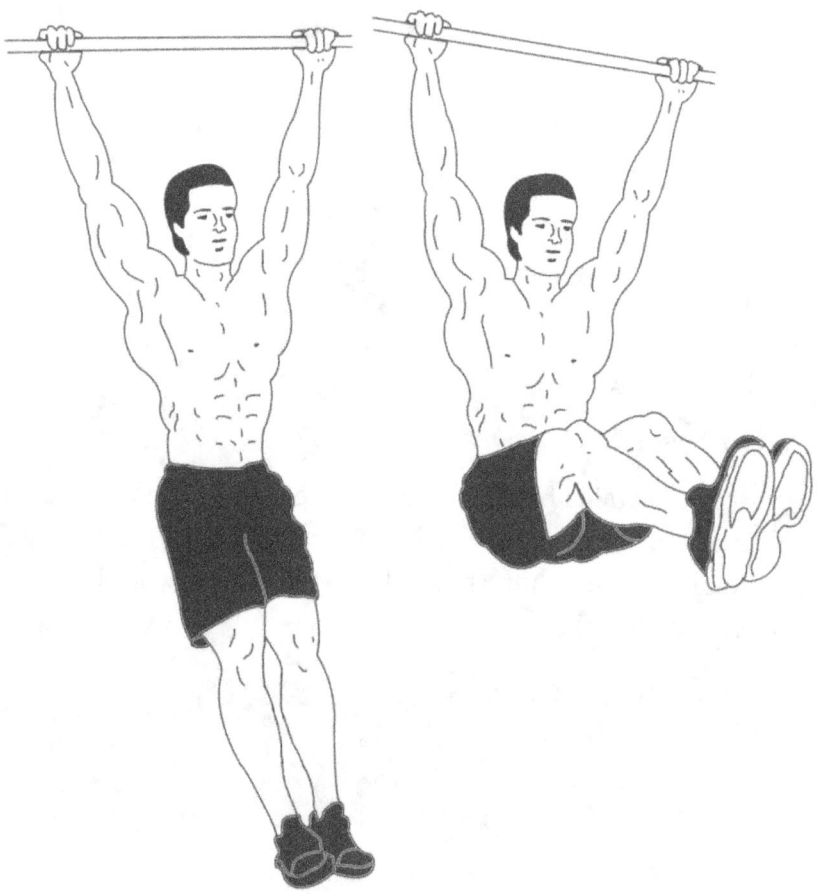

Level 7 Exercises

Toes to Bar/ HLL

Grip the Chin-Up bar, with your hands facing away from your body and a bit wider than shoulder width. Draw strength by bringing your feet up behind your body, swing forward and all the way up to the bar. Touch both feet to the bar and bring them back down.

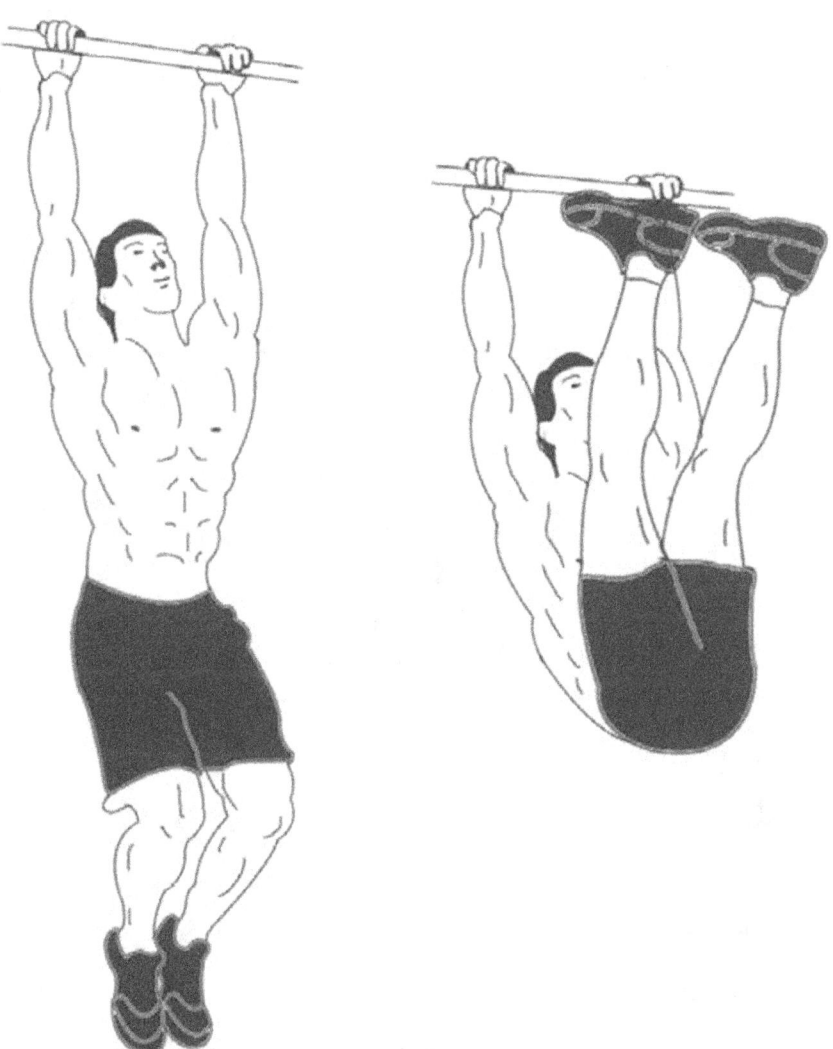

One-Legged Dragon Flag

Lie with your back flat against a bench, your arms raised and behind your head, grip the top of the bench. Bend one knee and tuck it against your bottom. In one effort, pull your body up and away from the bench- keep your whole body rigid and raise your torso until it is level with your shoulders, hold the position for 1 - 2 seconds and return your body slowly back down to the bench. Switch legs and repeat the above steps.

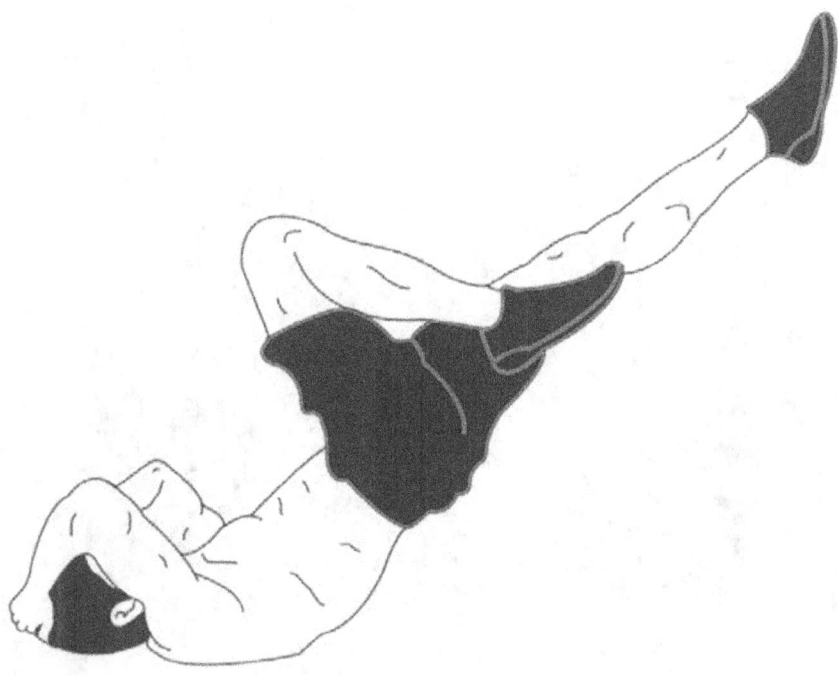

Level 8 Exercise

Dragon Flag

Lie with your back flat against a bench, your arms raised and behind your head, gripping the top of the bench. In one effort, pull your body up and away from the bench- keep your whole body rigid, and raise your torso until it is level with your shoulders, hold the position for 1 - 2 seconds and return your body slowly back down until your buttocks are an inch from the bench- do your repetitions without touching the bench.

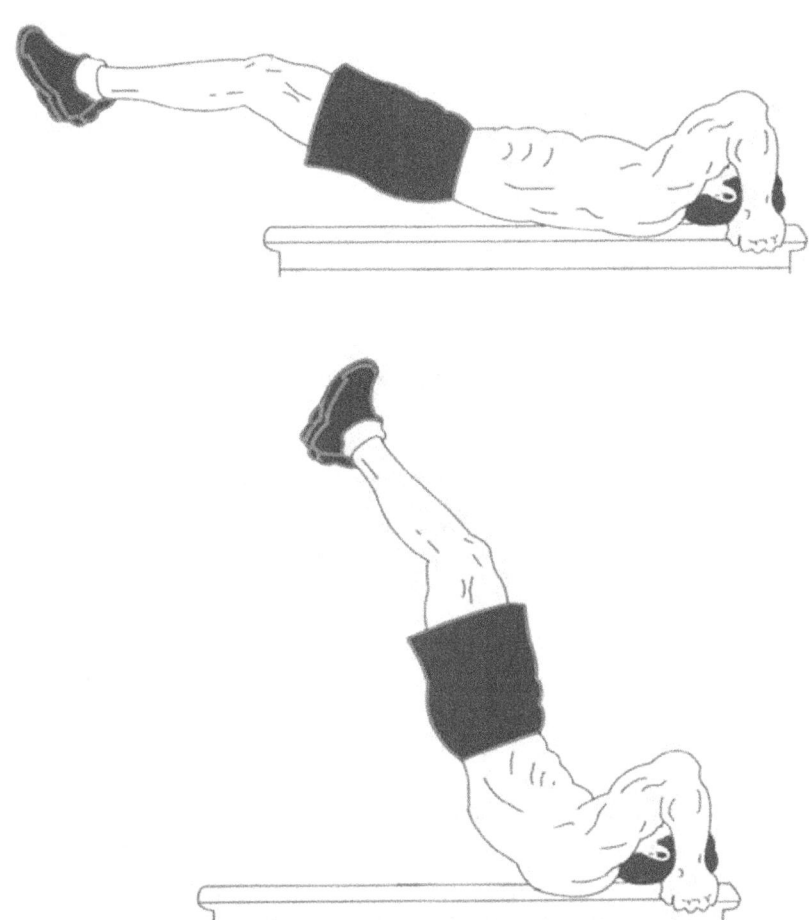

Level 9 Exercise

Dragon Variation Special Calisthenics 2.0

While doing a regular Dragon Flag, move your foot as if you were swimming.

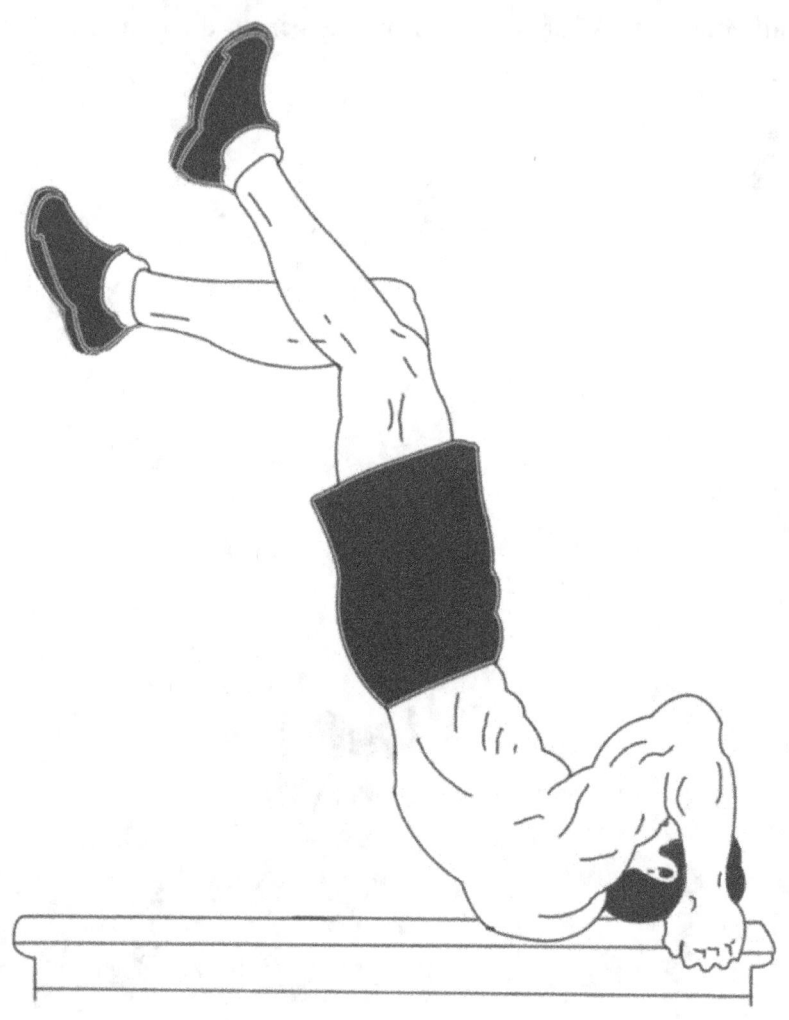

Obliques

Level 1 Exercises

Russian Twist

Sit down on an exercise mat. (For added intensity, you can hold a medicine ball here- hold it with both hands.) Bend your knees slightly and lift your feet off the ground. Lean back approx. 30

degrees, and hold yourself up using your abs. Twist your body to the left with the medicine ball, and twist it to the right with the medicine ball.

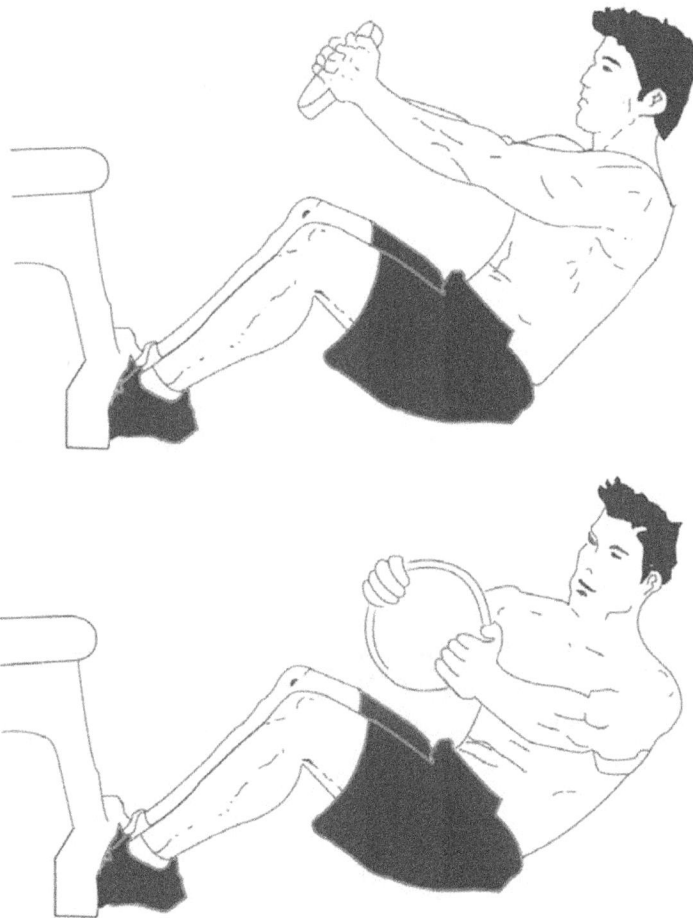

Side Plank

Lie down on a mat, with your left side against it. Make sure your feet are together, on top of each other. Using your forearm and elbow, prop yourself up. Raise your hips and hold this position for 2 seconds. Repeat for your right side.

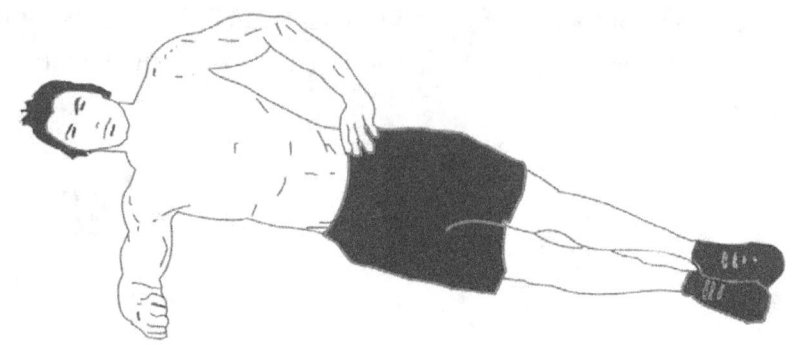

Level 2 Exercises

Mountain Climber

Place your body in a Push-Up position, arms fully extended. Lift your right foot and bring your knee to your chest. Do this as close as possible. Touch your foot to the ground and repeat for the opposite leg.

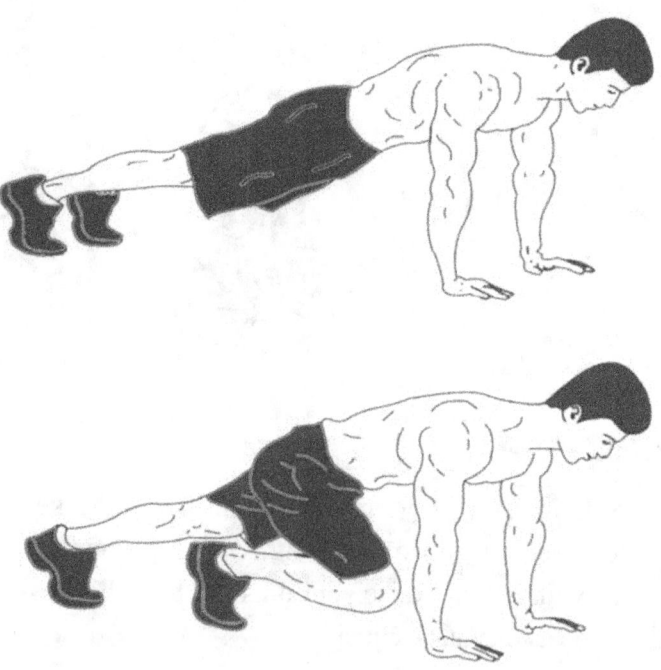

Level 3 Exercises

Foot to Foot Crunches

Lie on the ground, with your hands at your sides, knees bent and feet flat on the ground. Raise your head, tighten your abs, and stretch your hands to your heels. Hold this position for 2 - 4 seconds. Repeat crunches without letting your back touch the ground.

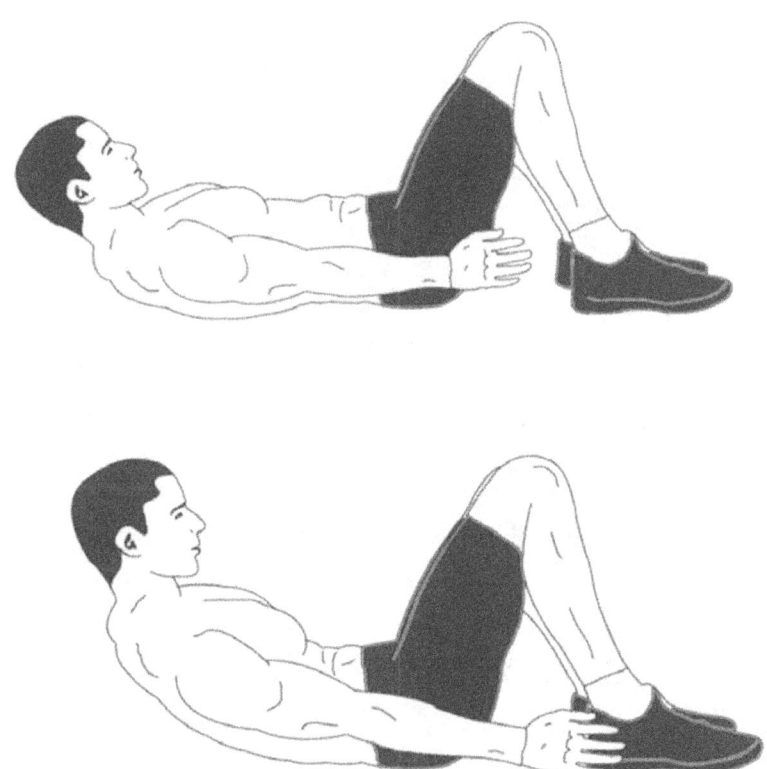

Bicycle Crunch

Lie down on the floor, with your hands behind your head and your legs straight. Bend your knees. Raise your left leg up to your chest and raise your head at the same time, twisting to the same side your knee is pulled up to your chest, keep your hands behind your head. Switch legs and repeat the above steps.

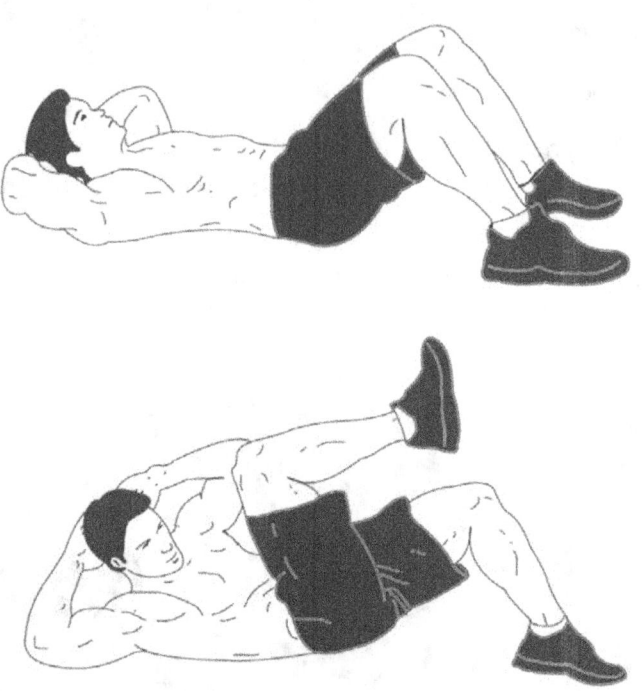

Single-Leg Side Plank

Lie on your left side on a mat and place your feet sideways on top of each other. Use your left forearm and left elbow to prop yourself up. Place your right hand on your hip and raise your right leg high, as high as you can. Raise your hips and hold it for 30 seconds. Lower yourself back down. Switch sides and repeat the above steps.

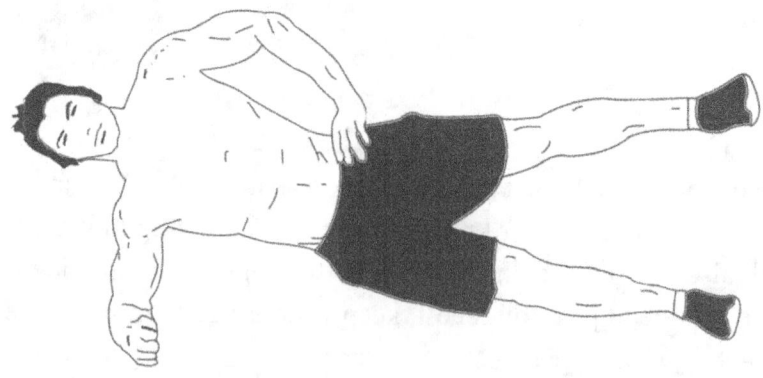

Level 4 Exercise

Declined Foot to Foot Crunches

Same steps for the foot to foot crunch, except you will be performing it on a declined bench.

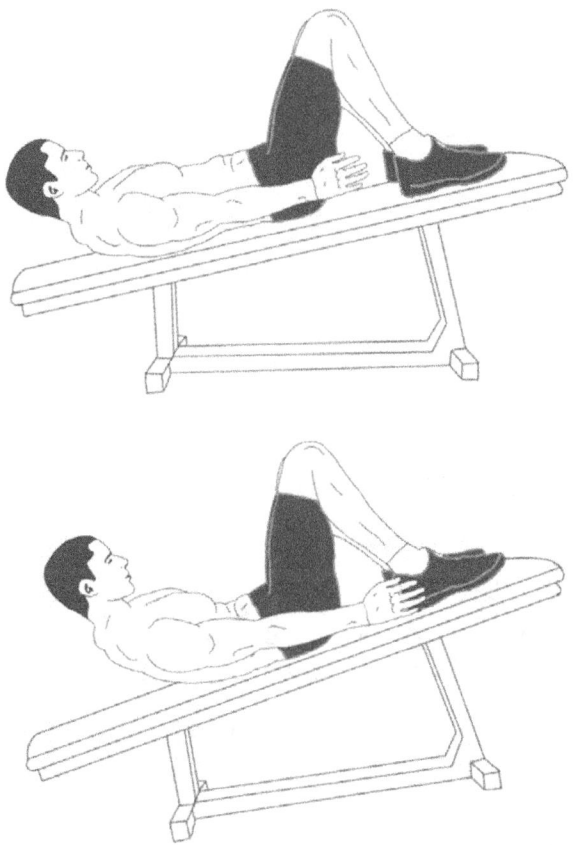

Level 5 Exercises

Hanging-Knee Raised-Oblique Crunch/ Corkscrew

Grip a horizontal bar, lining your feet straight under your body, with your hands a bit wider than your shoulder width. Tighten your abs and raise your knees to your chest, while twisting your body to your left side then right side.

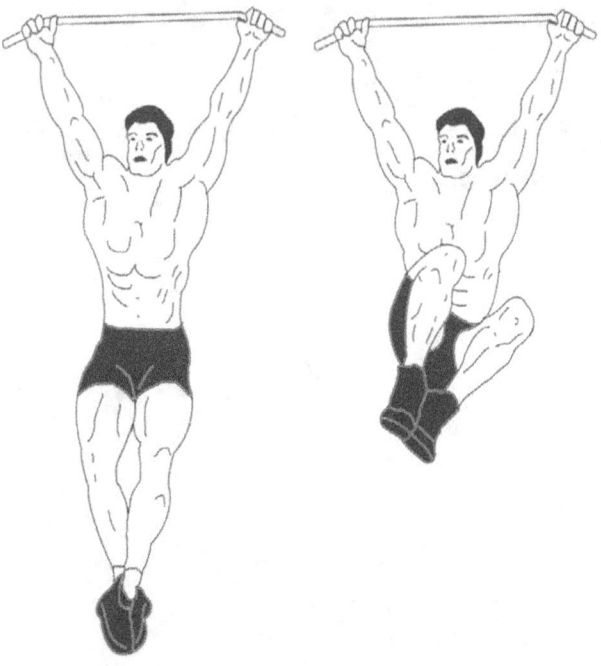

Side-Oblique Crunches

Lie on your right side and place your legs on top of each other. Bend your knees a little and place your left hand at the back of your head. Proceed by performing a crunch, except this time sideways, as we are focusing on your oblique muscles. Repeat on the other side.

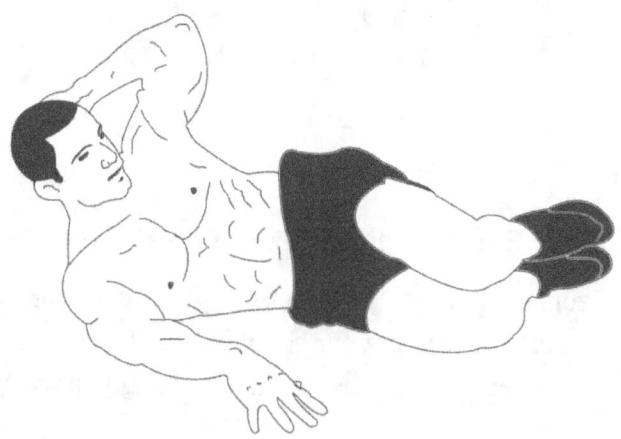

Level 6 Exercise

Hanging Corkscrews

Grip a horizontal bar and make sure your legs are hanging straight. Contract your muscles and pull your legs up and to the right. Repeat one side three more times, then do the other side.

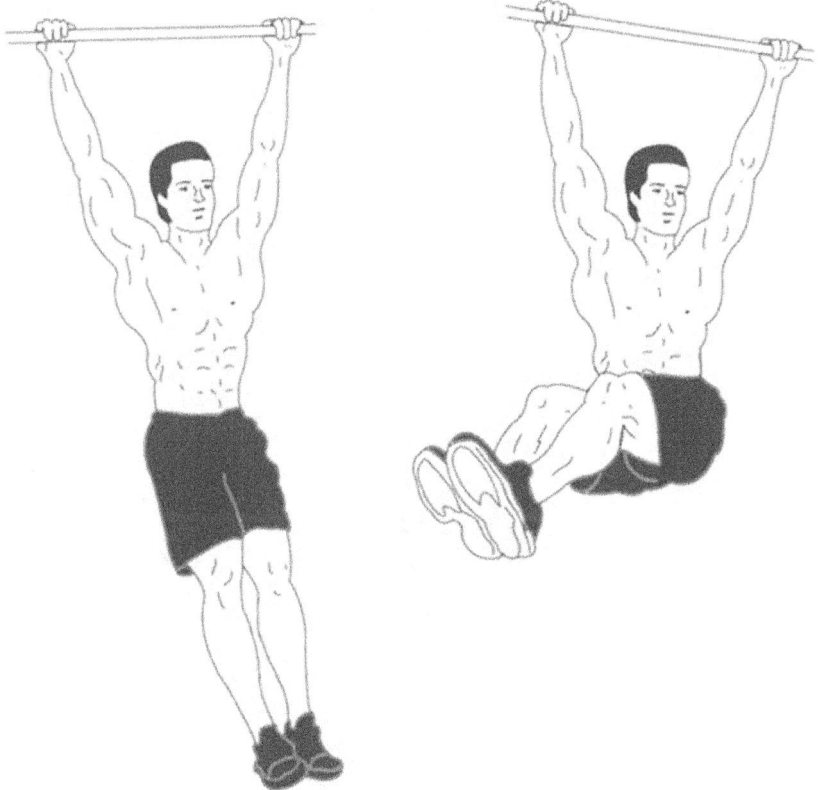

Level 7 Exercise

Hanging Windshield Wipers

Grip a pull-up bar and raise your legs until they are parallel to the ground. Tense your abs, rotate your legs to the right as far as you can, then rotate to the other side.

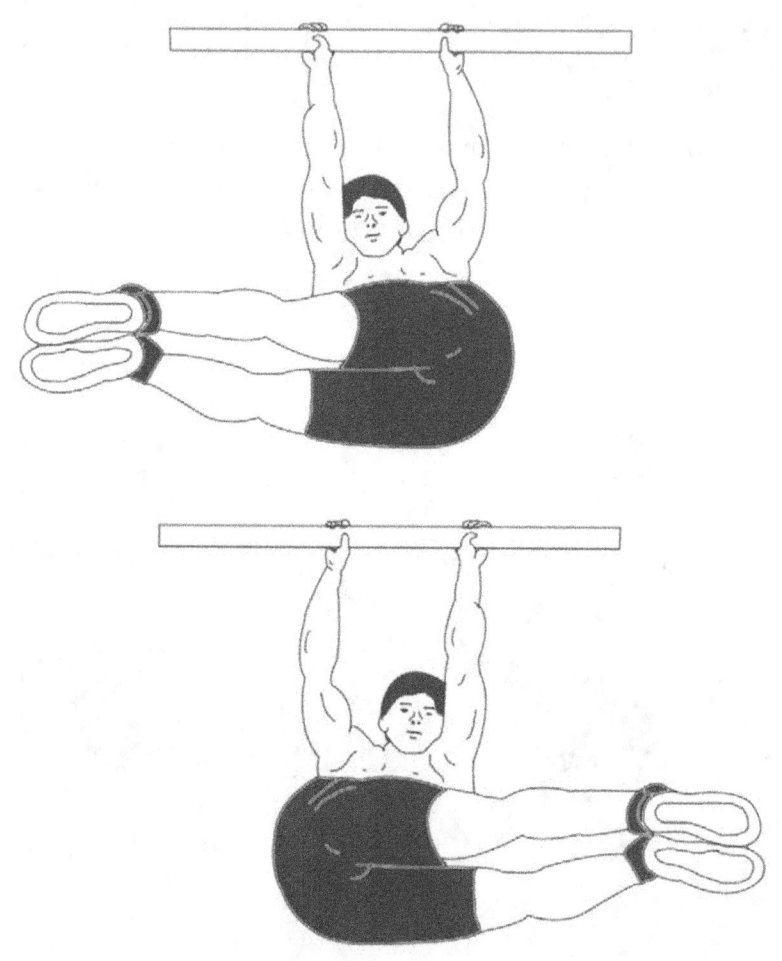

Triceps

Level 1 Exercise

Triceps Extension On The Wall (Ultimate, Newbie Exercise)

The full name for the triceps muscle worked in this exercise is referred to as the *Triceps Brachii*. It is the muscle at the back of your arms, and its primary purpose is to align your arms appropriately.

It is critical to extend the triceps and warm up before you attempt this exercise; some cardio to raise your heart rate.

Lastly, it is crucial to maintain suppleness of your muscles so your body recovers from the workout. These extends should be held for no less than ten seconds.

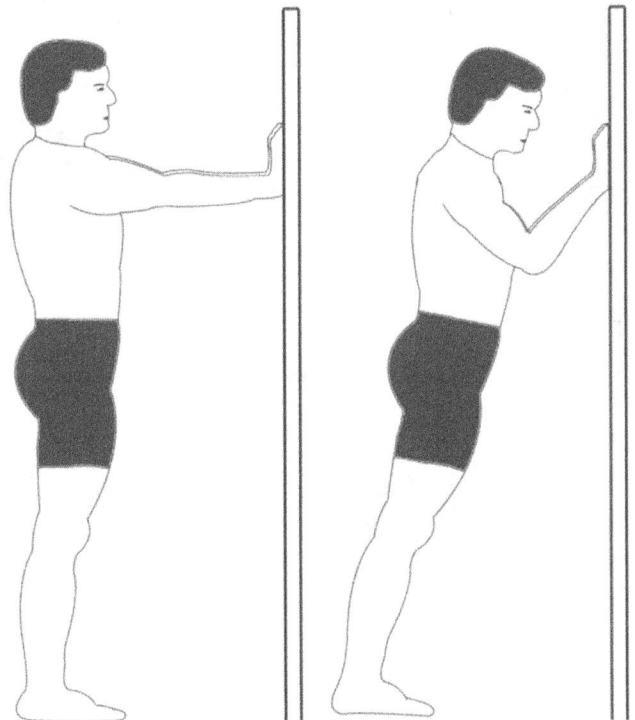

Steps to Follow:

Step 1: Stand with your right side placed against a wall.

Step 2: Raise your right arm above your body, rest your elbow at a slightly acute angle against the wall.

Step 3: Lean toward the divider. Feel the stretch in your right tricep.

Step 4: Switch sides. Repeat the process.

Level 2 Exercises

Triceps Extension on Knees

Place your body in normal "Push-Up On Knees" position on the floor, but place your hands a bit higher than your shoulders. Lower yourself to your forearms, really focus on the extension back up, to isolate the triceps and not work the shoulders and chest, like the basic Push-Up.

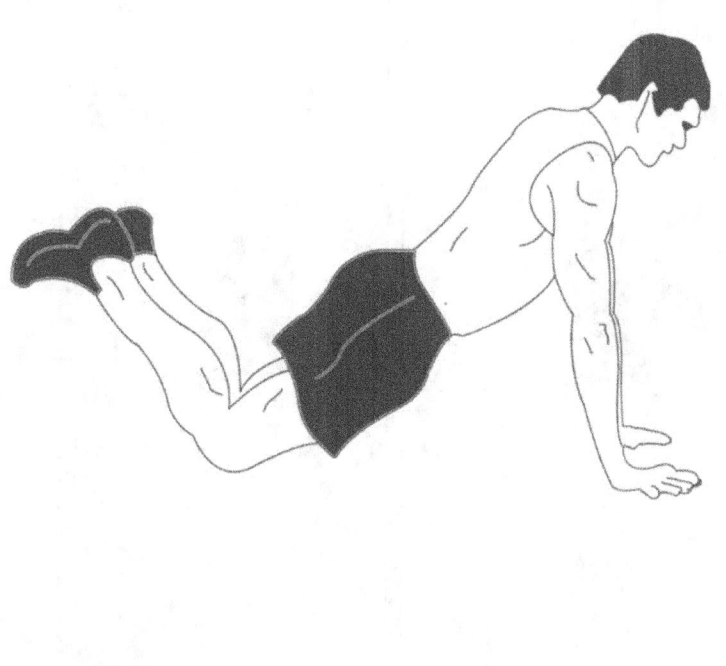

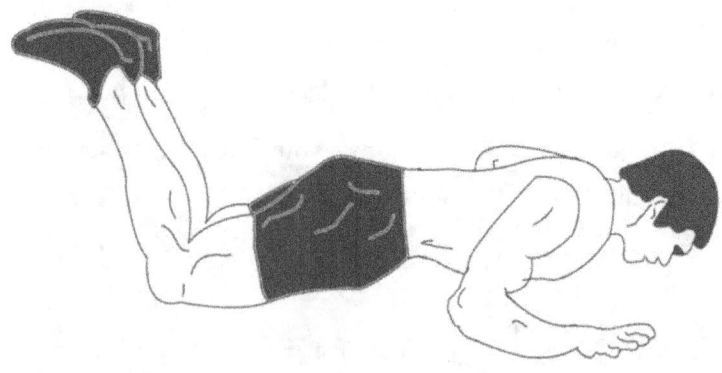

Diamond Push-Up On Knees

This particular Push-Up is used often as a warm-up exercise, as part of the Army's exercising tactics.

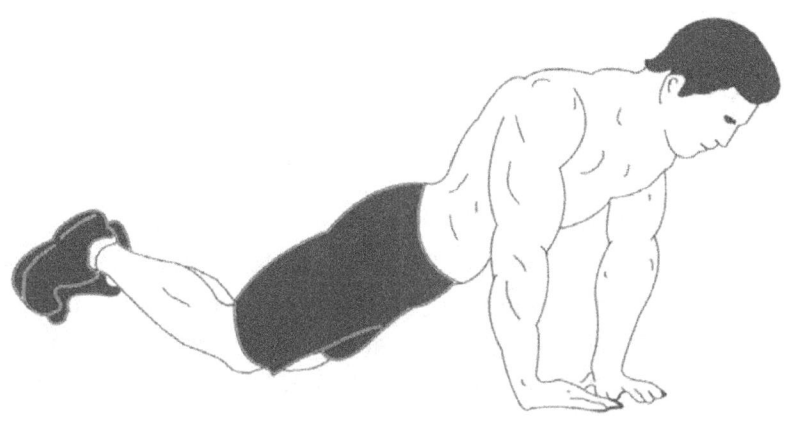

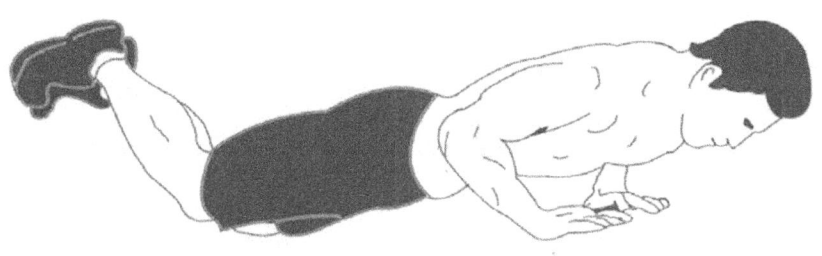

Steps to Follow:

Step 1: Lie inclined on floor with your hands wider than shoulder width. While maintaining bent knees, raise your body from the floor by extending your arms, and keeping your back straight.

Step 2: Return to the ground by bending your arms.

Step 3: Elevate your body upwards by pushing your arms until they are completely extended.

Additional Information

Both the upper and the lower body parts must be kept straight throughout the entire process. You forefeet should maintain their pose on the floor, as your body rotates on its knees.

Level 3 Exercise

Triceps-Bar Extension (Elbows Facing Down)

Grip weights with both hands and position your feet apart, lined up under your hips. Lift the weights over our head and fully extend your arms. Keep your elbows tight against your body and increase the resistance by doing a semicircular motion behind your head. Do this until you touch your forearms with your Biceps.

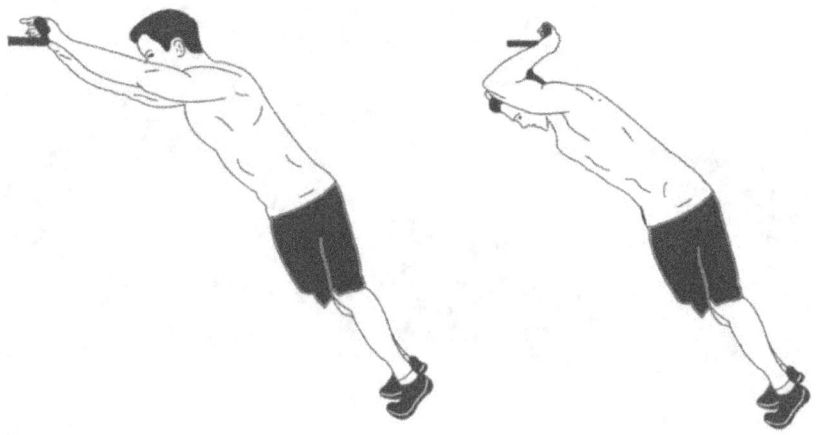

Level 4 Exercise

Diamond Push-Up

Get yourself into the classic Push-Up position, placing your forefingers and thumbs in a diamond formation. Tuck your abs and lower your body, perform a Push-Up. Maintain the diamond position with your hands.

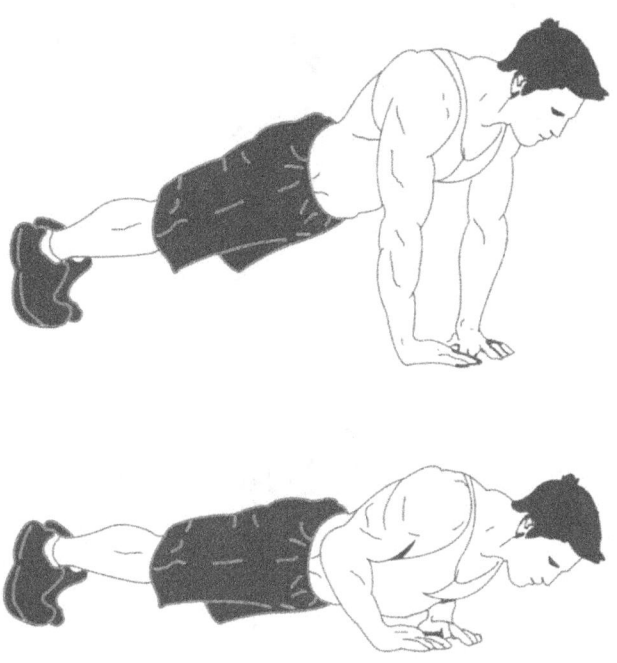

Level 5 Exercise

Forearm to Triceps Extension Push-Up

Steps to Follow:

Step 1: Assume a typical push up position with both elbows perpendicularly bent against the ground and angled sideways, your lower arms should assume a parallel pose to the ground. The right hand should be in contact with the left elbow, while the left hand should be in contact with the right elbow, to delineate the shape of a trapezium of sorts.

Step 2: Elevate your body up from the floor by stretching your forearms keeping your body straight. Push your body up until forearms are fully extended.

Step 3: Lower your body to floor by bending your arms until you return to starting pose.

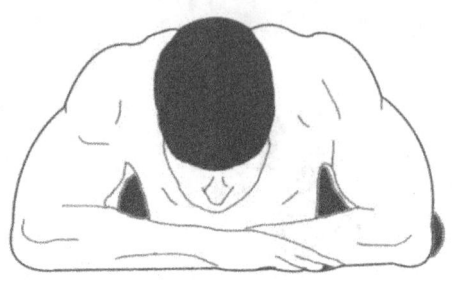

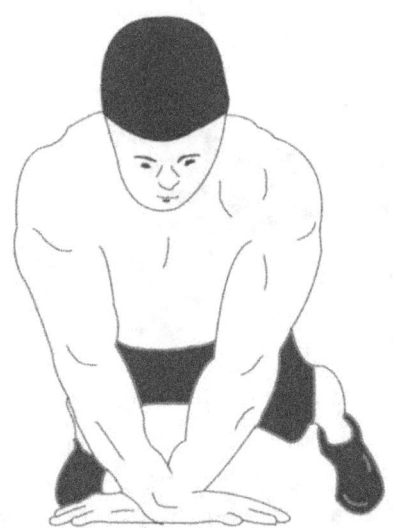

Level 6 Exercise

Closed-Grips Straight Bar Dips

This is one of the most difficult dip variations. Try not to chip away at it, until you can do no less than ten back-to-back dips on the parallel bar.

As the name proposes, this activity is performed with both hands set together, with a closed grip on the straight bar. Your grip should be closed and you will begin to notice how tough it is after a while.

Steps to Follow:

Step 1: When you dip on a straight bar, your body must shift around the bar. As you lower yourself down, you will have to hang over the bar and stretch your legs out a bit to maintain your balance. This action brings about additional abdominal intensity while demanding more from the shoulders.

Step 2: Lower yourself all the way down when you are dipping on the straight bar. Your midsection or chest should touch the bar, creating the same perpendicular angle at the outside of your elbows, at the base of every rep.

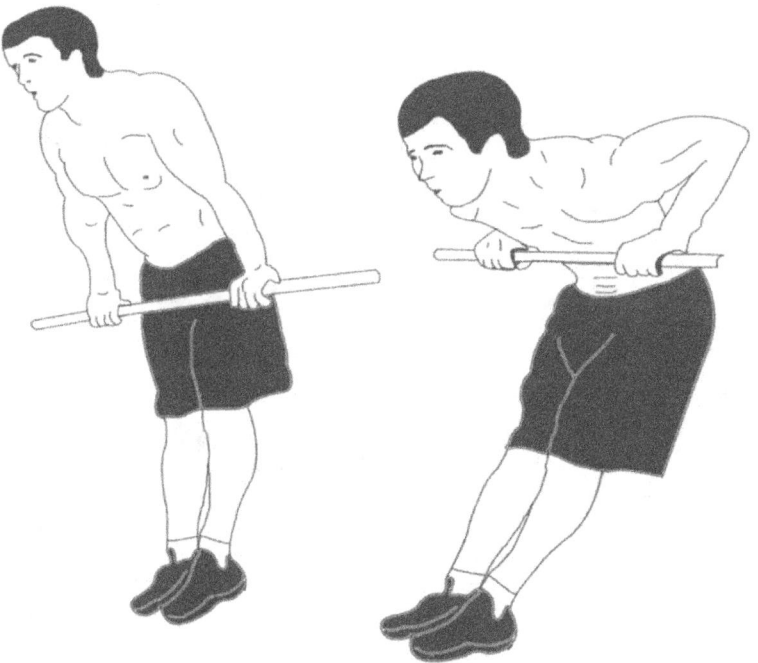

Additional Information

Try not to let your shoulders shrug as you lower your body, focus that your arms don't flare out. Ensure your elbows point behind you, at the bottom of the rep.

Level 7 Exercise

Triceps Extensions Push-Up

Place your body in normal Push-Up position on the floor, placing your hands a bit higher than your shoulders. Lower your body to your forearms, really focus on the extension back up, to isolate the triceps and not work the shoulders and chest, like the basic Push-Up.

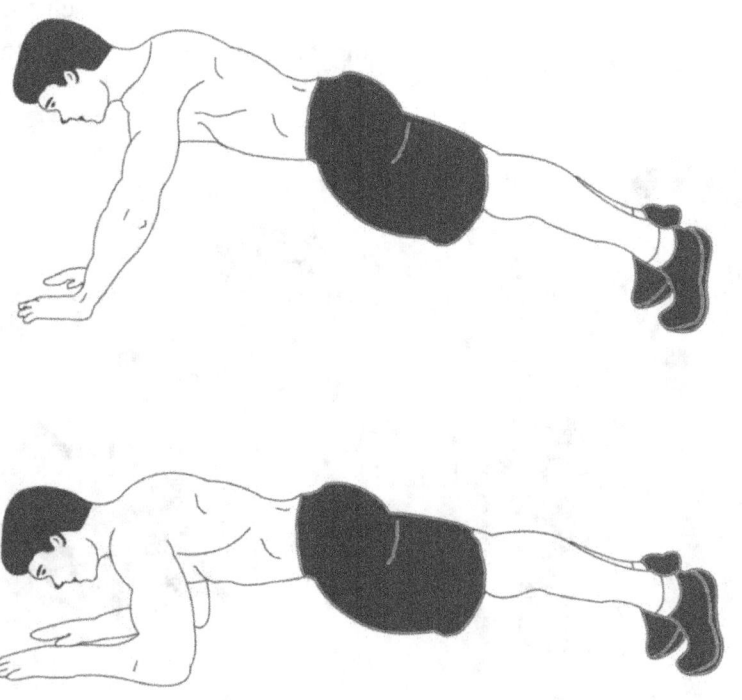

Level 8 Exercise

Russian Dip

Russian Dips principally work three muscle ranges: wrists, shoulders, and triceps. Drilling Russian plunges has a huge carryover impact for performing a muscle-up. I am referring to a genuine muscle-up. This drill will obviously help with the muscle-up extensively. Be that as it may, if you are looking to really develop your gymnastic muscle-up, then these dips should be a staple activity in your daily exercise routine.

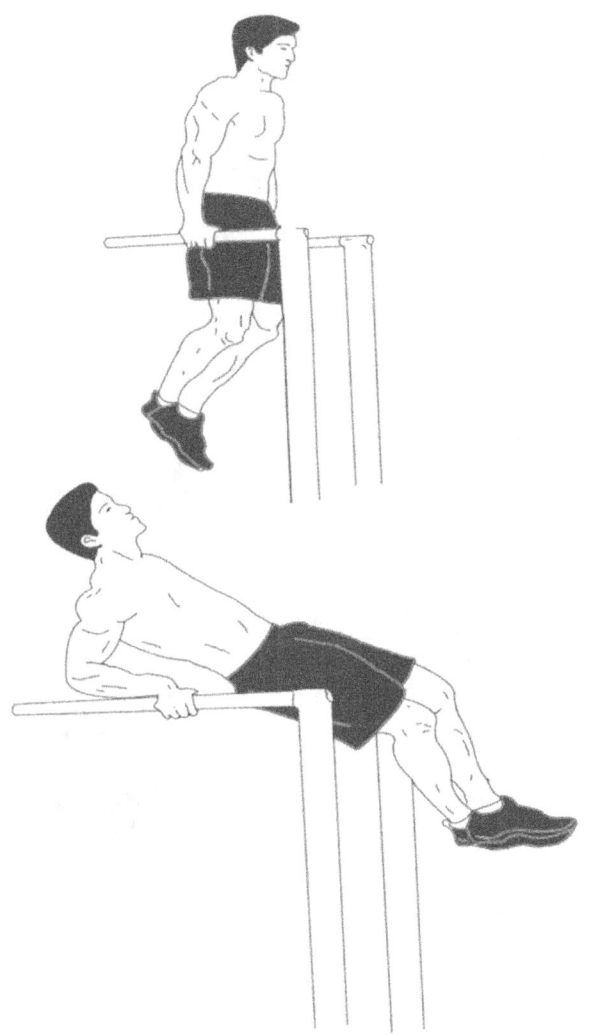

Steps to Follow:

Russian dip is a gymnastics drill, executed on parallel bars and considered to be one of the hardest dips or plunges variations.

Step 1: Place your lower arms against the parallel bars, while suspending your body in the air, maintain an upward stance.

Step 2: Maintain your arms in the top dip position, as your hands support your body.

Level 9 Exercise

Regular HSPU (Handstand Push-Up) (Free/Against Wall)

This handstand Push-Up is an amazing workout for your triceps, where you force down your full body weight from a reversed position.

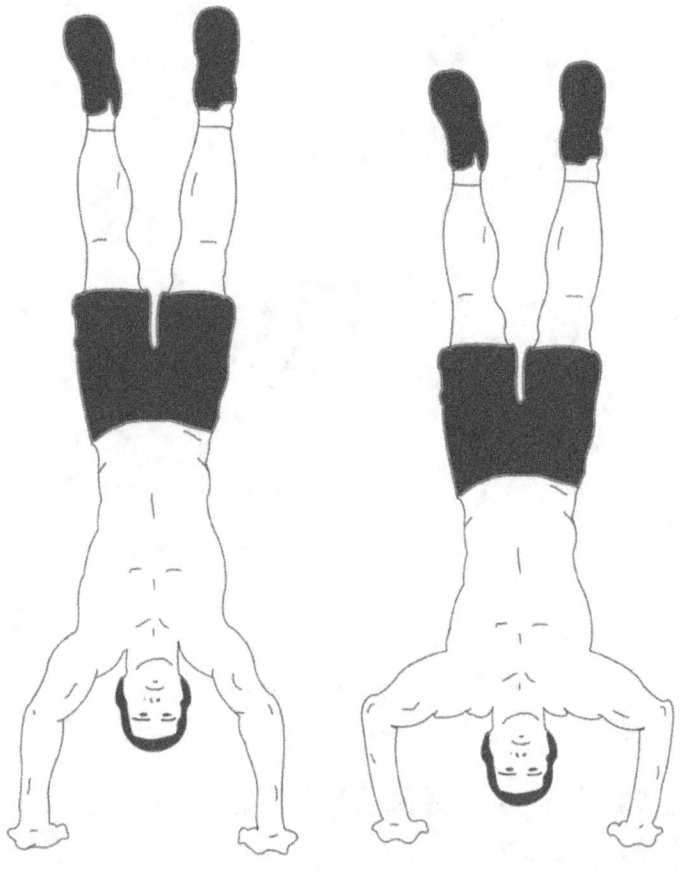

Steps to Follow:

The position to observe when practicing this activity; bent at hips, with your hands on the floor a few inches from the wall.

Step 1: Place your palms a bit wider than shoulder width, on the ground, about two steps away from the wall.

Step 2: Kneel with one leg under your body, place it just below your rib-cage.

Step 3: Extend your other leg behind you. Keep this leg completely straight.

Step 4: Press up, with the leg under you.

Step 5: Swerve the trailing leg up; the back leg will do the majority of the work.

Additional Information

Apart from the undeniable intensity of this exercise:

1. It creates mind blowing shoulder and abdominal strength.

2. It is amazing for balance training.

3. It helps strengthen your glutes and core.

Level 10 Exercise

Diamond HSPU (Diamond Grip Handstand Push-Up)

Place your hands on the floor, a bit wider than shoulder width, in a diamond formation; forefingers and thumbs touching. Make sure there is a wall near, so you can do a handstand with your back facing away from the wall, and your feet placed flat against it. Do a Push-Up while in this position.

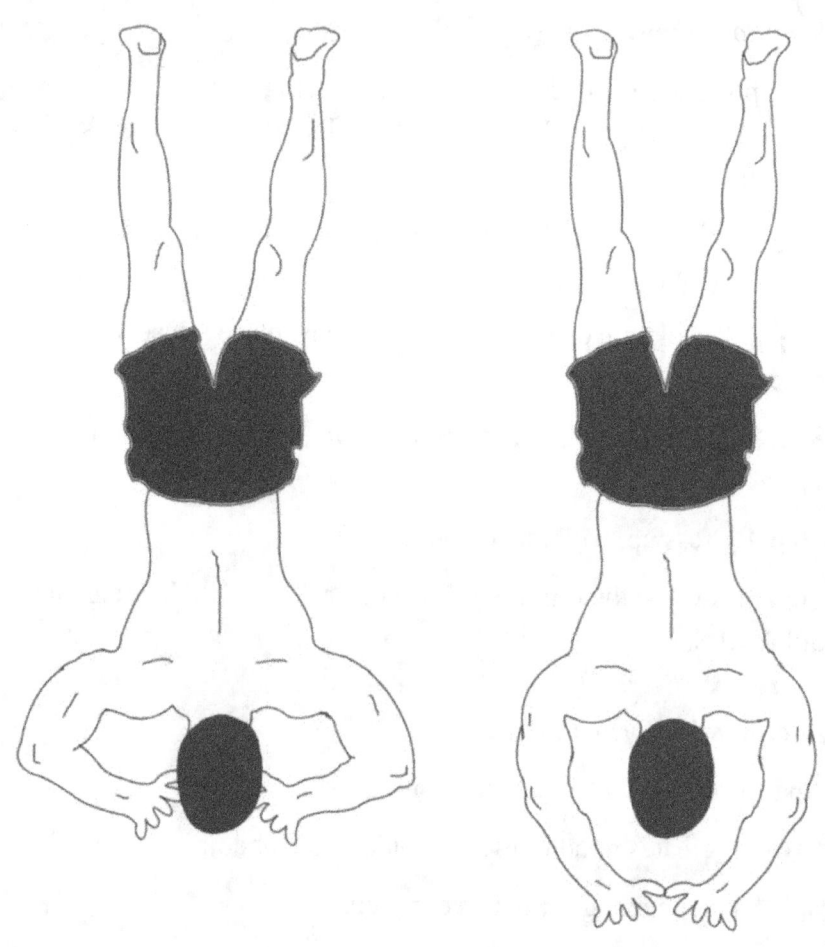

Back

Level 1 Exercise

Pull-Up Negative

Stand on a platform and grip the bar, palms facing away from your body. Pull your body up and over, until your chin passes the bar. Repeat Pull-Ups without touching the ground.

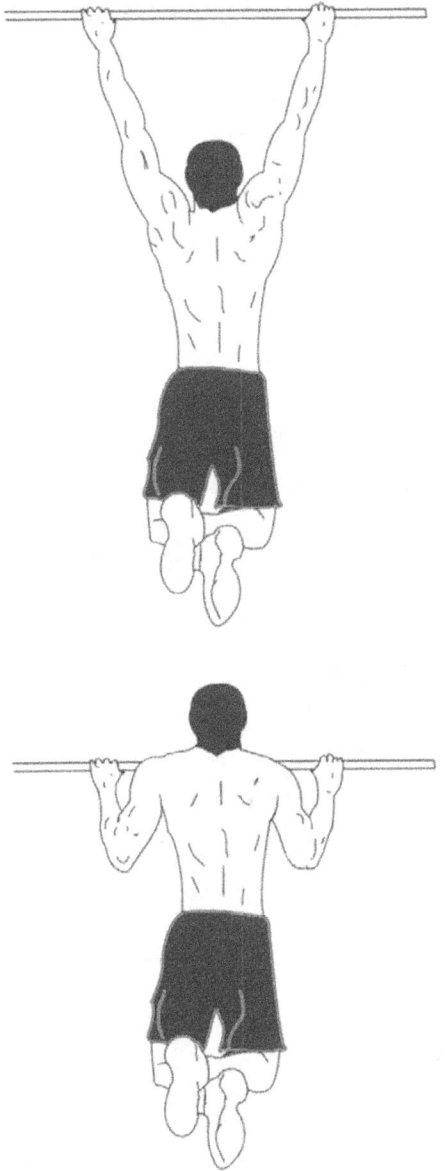

Hip-Up

Lie on your back, on the floor. Your hands should be on your sides, palms facing down. Keep your knees bent and your feet flat on the floor. Lift your lower back or buttocks, your upper back should remain pressed to the floor. Do this while you are squeezing your buttocks and push your hips high up in the air, as high as you can. Keep pushing until your hips and knees are almost aligned and hold this position for 2 - 4 seconds. Lower your body back to the floor.

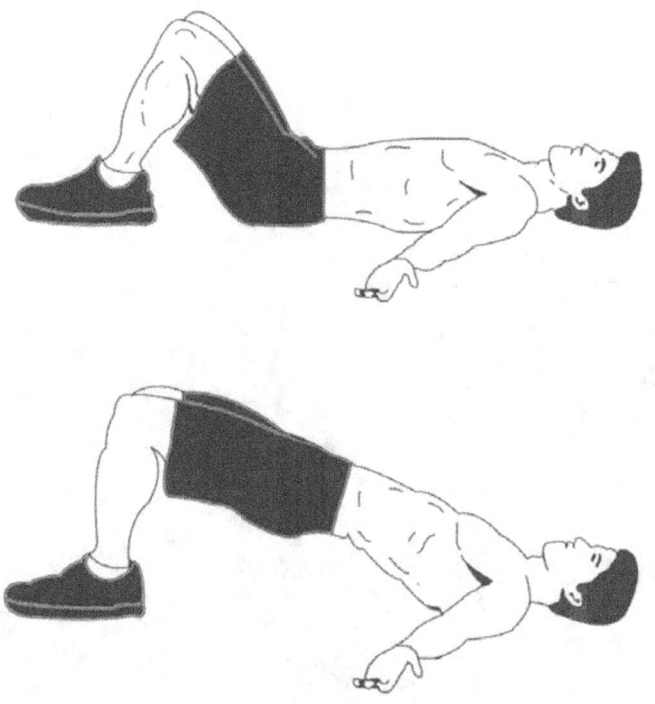

Level 2 Exercises

Hanging Row (Chest almost to bar)

Lie on the floor beneath the bar. Wrap your hands around the bar, palms facing away from your body. Tighten your core and pull yourself up until your chest touches the bar. Repeat without touching the ground.

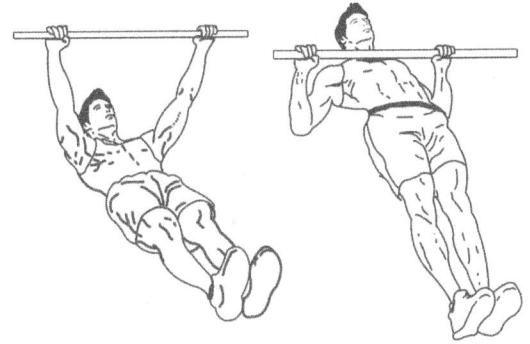

Superman (stay in position for 3 seconds = 1 repetition)

Lie on the mat face down, legs fully extended. Raise your arms, legs, and chest for 2 – 4 seconds while exhaling. Then inhale and lower your legs, arms, and chest back down.

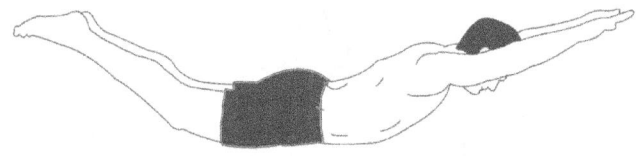

Level 3 Exercises

Pronated-Grip Pull-Up

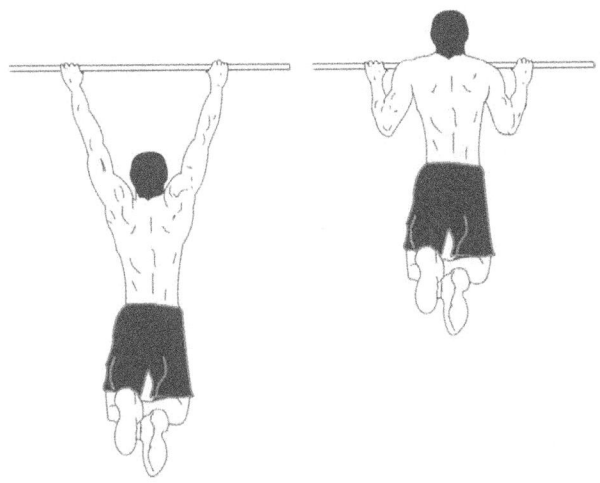

Level 4 Exercise

Side to Side/Diagonal Pull-Up

Grab the horizontal bar, palms facing away from your body with your hands a bit wider than shoulder width. Pull your body up while directing your chin over your left hand, then immediately over your right hand.

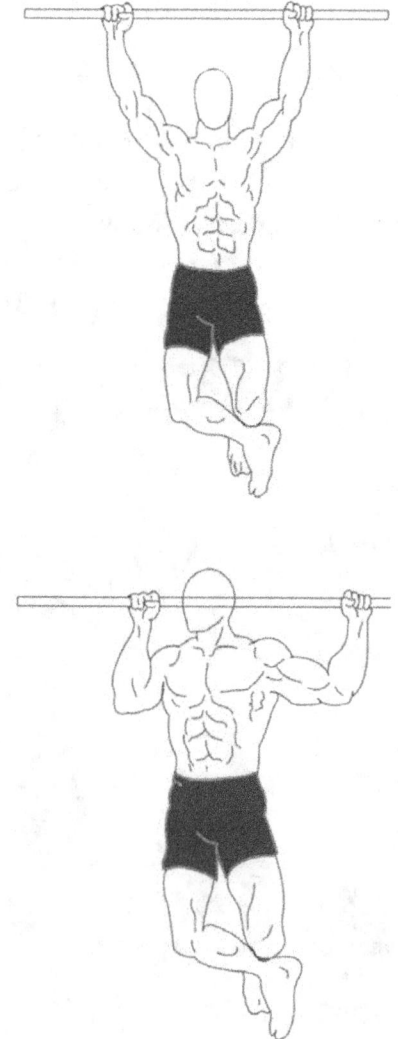

Level 5 Exercise

Sternum Pull-Up Bar (chest to bar)

This exercise is just like your basic Pull-Up, instead of your chin passing the bar, you need to pull your body up high enough so your chest is even with the bar.

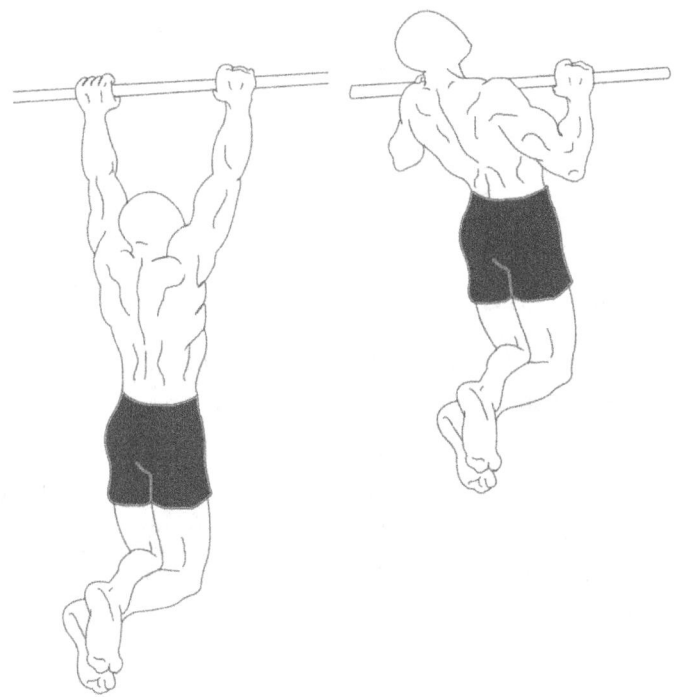

Level 6 Exercises

Muscle-Up Pull

Hold the bar using a false grip. (False grip is your thumb on top of the bar, not around it.) Pull your body up and over the bar, then press your hands down while you are driving your body up to make a dip. This movement works your chest, your arms, forearms and shoulders, but also your back. It has been included here as it's a movement you must master.

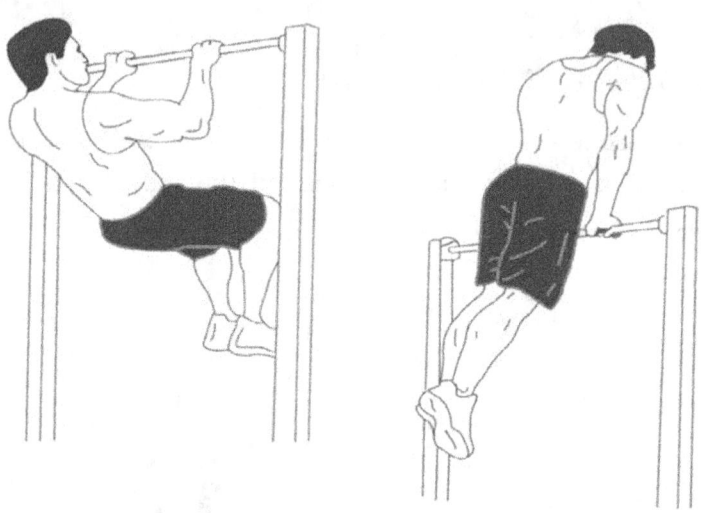

One-Leg Back Lever

You are probably aware of the exercise 'skin the cat,' this is an important exercise for this lever. Once you are at this position, lower your body until your back is parallel with the ground while keeping one knee up to your chest. Hold this position as long as you can. You may start with the tucked back lever. For additional information, check the bonus bank of exercises, in which I explain levers in details.

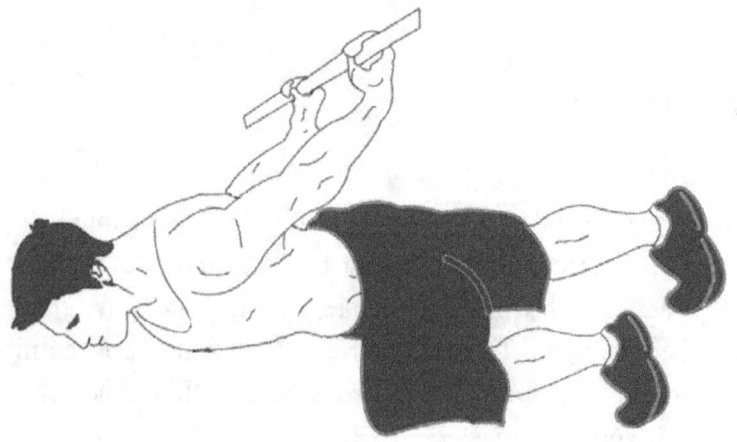

Stall Bar RLL

Lie on the ground, with your back flat and arms extended above your head. Make sure there is a bar you can grip above your head. Now, slowly raise both your legs, hips and lower back without bending them. Yours shoulder should remain flat on the ground. Repeat without touching the ground.

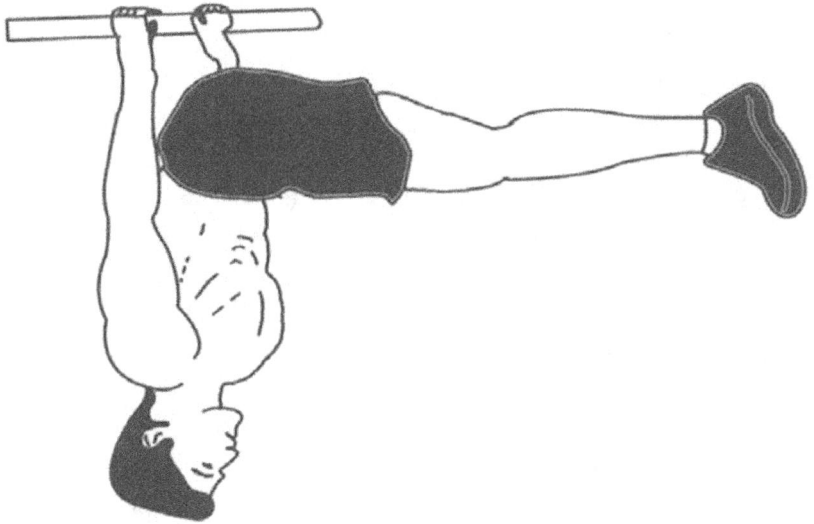

Level 7 Exercises

Hanging L-Sit Row

Pressing your back against the wall, gripping rings. Pulling your elbows against your body, and maintaining a straight back, pull your lower body up and perform an L-Sit.

Back Lever

Perform the *skin the cat* exercise while gripping a horizontal bar.

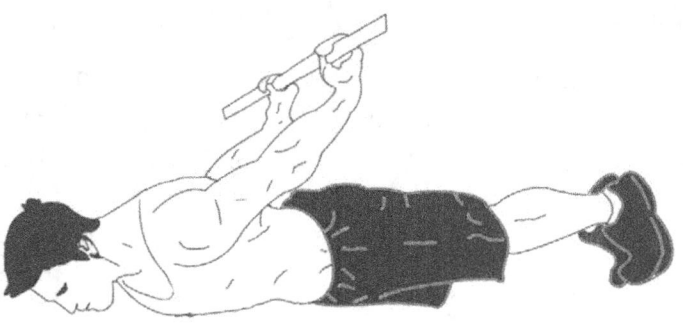

Level 8 Exercise

Back Lever Special Calisthenics 2.0

While doing the back lever, keep your upper body straight and move your legs to your left and then to the right (1 repetition).

Legs

Level 1 Exercise

Squats

Stand up with your feet apart. Step a bit forward, placing your feet shoulder width apart. Make sure your head is up, inhale and bend your knees in a squat position. Exhale and stand back up.

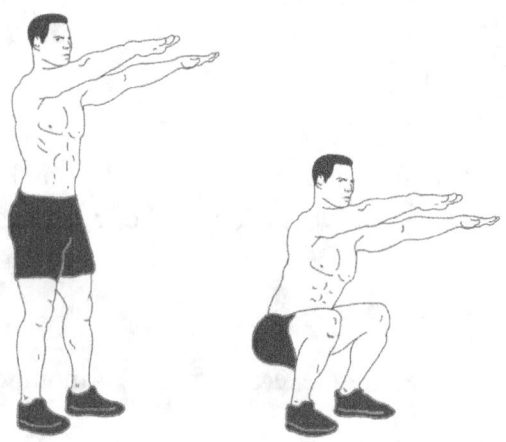

Level 2 Exercises

Wall Sit (2sec = 1rep)

Stand up with your back against a wall, placing your feet half a foot away from the wall. Your arms should be at your sides. Bend your knees and lower your body until your thighs become parallel to the floor. Hold for 2 seconds.

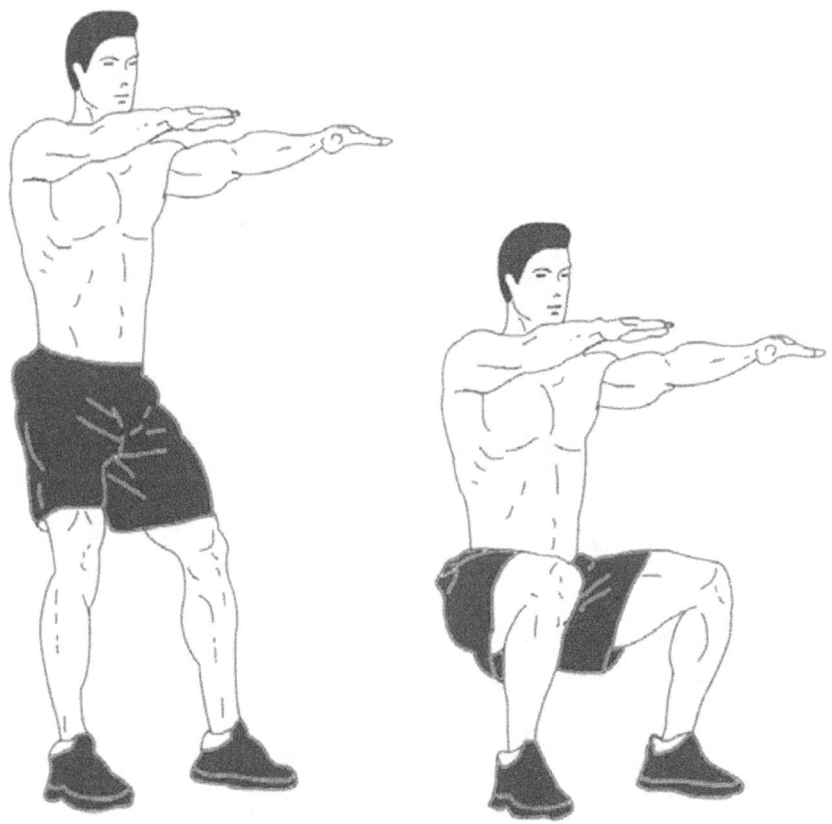

Box Jumps

Stand straight in front of a box. Squat down in a jumping motion. Jump onto the box and thrust your arms in the air.

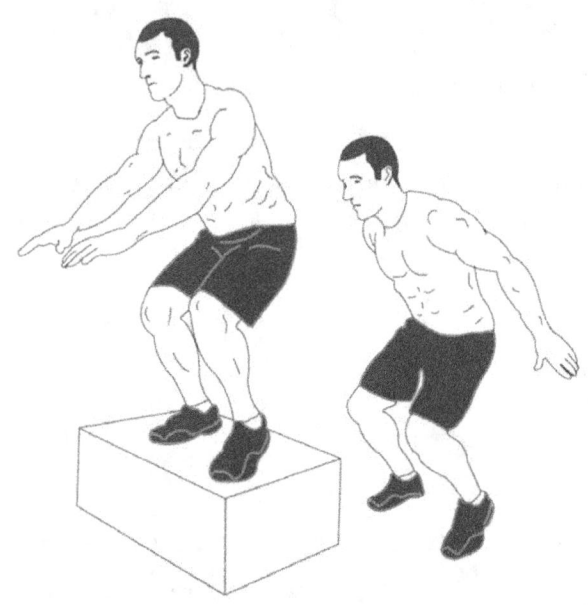

Calf Raises

Using resistance bands in both hands, bring them up to your shoulders and stand up. Line your feet under your hips. Raise your toes as high as you can and back down to the ground.

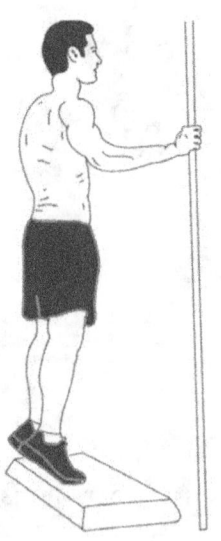 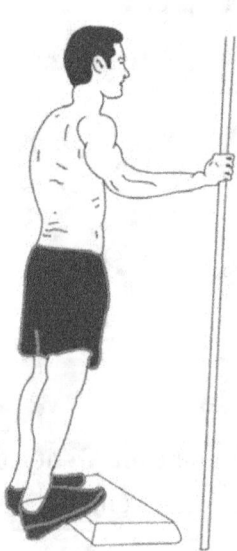

Level 3 Exercise

Lunge

Start off with one leg in front, the other behind. Make sure you have enough space in between your legs so that one leg is not on top of the other. Lunge straight down. Your shoulders are rolled back. Your chest and abs are tight. You're going to keep the weight in your front heel. Lunge straight down, dropping your back knee to the floor until it almost touch it. Go back and repeat.

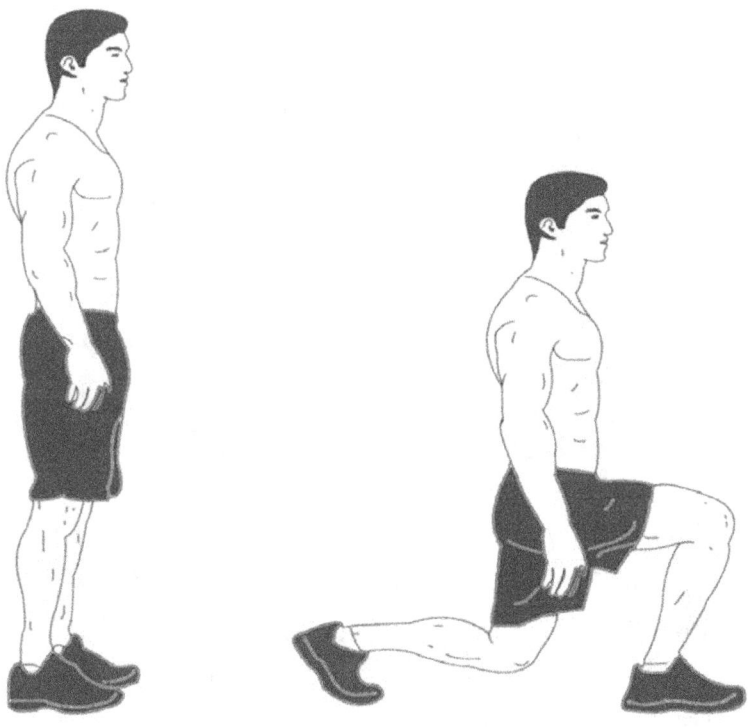

Level 4 Exercises

One-Leg Calf Raise

You can use a weight plate or step for this exercise. For beginners who need balance, you can hold onto a wall. Place your toes at the edge of the plate/step. Lift one leg up, and press your ankle of the lifted leg, against that back of your calf. Push up on the toes of your other foot, maintaining a straight back and balance. Lower back down. Switch legs, repeat the steps above.

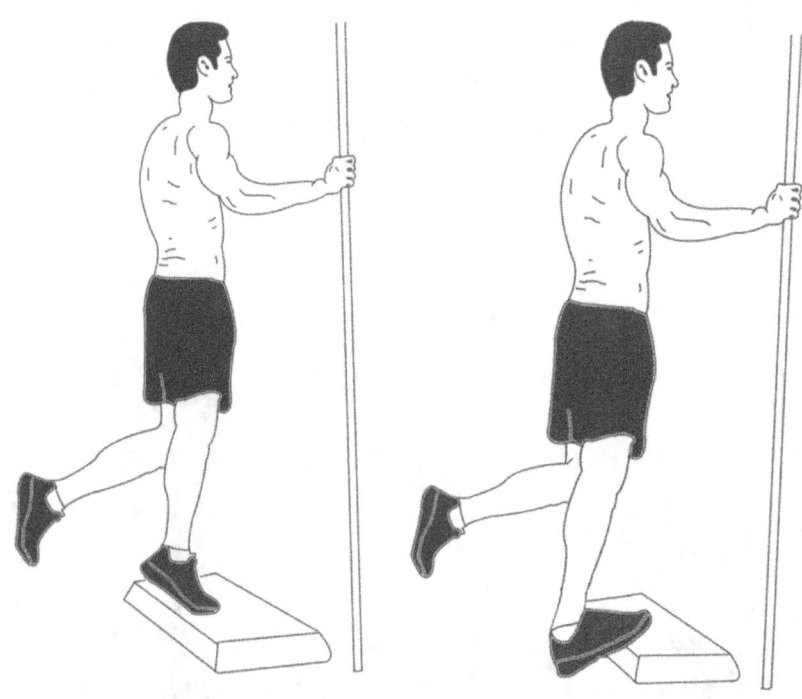

Wall Sit (4sec = 1rep)

Stand up with your back against a wall, placing your feet half a foot away from the wall. Your arms should be at your sides. Bend your knees and lower your body until your thighs become parallel to the floor. Hold for 4 seconds.

Level 5 Exercise

Wall Sit (6sec = 1rep)

Stand up with your back against a wall, placing your feet half a foot away from the wall. Your arms should be at your sides. Bend your knees and lower your body until your thighs become parallel to the floor. Hold for 4 seconds.

Single Leg Wall Sit (2sec = 1rep)

Stand up with your back against a wall, placing your feet half a foot away from the wall. Your arms should be at your sides. Bend your knees and lower your body until your thighs become parallel to the floor. Form an 'L' with one leg. Hold for 2 seconds. Stay as long as needed and then do the same with the other leg.

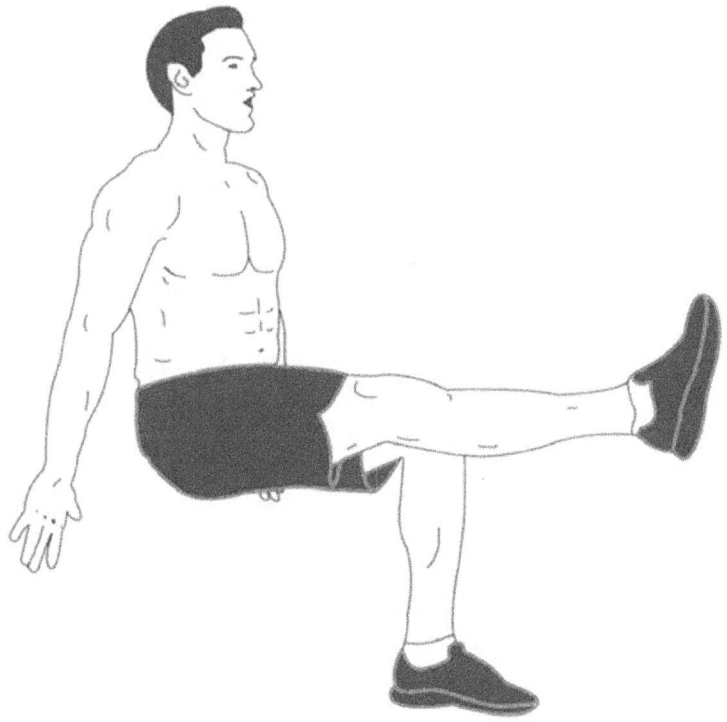

Single Leg Burpee

Place your body in a Push-Up position. Perform a Push-Up, kick your foot back into your hands, jump in the air while raising your hands. Repeat on the other side.

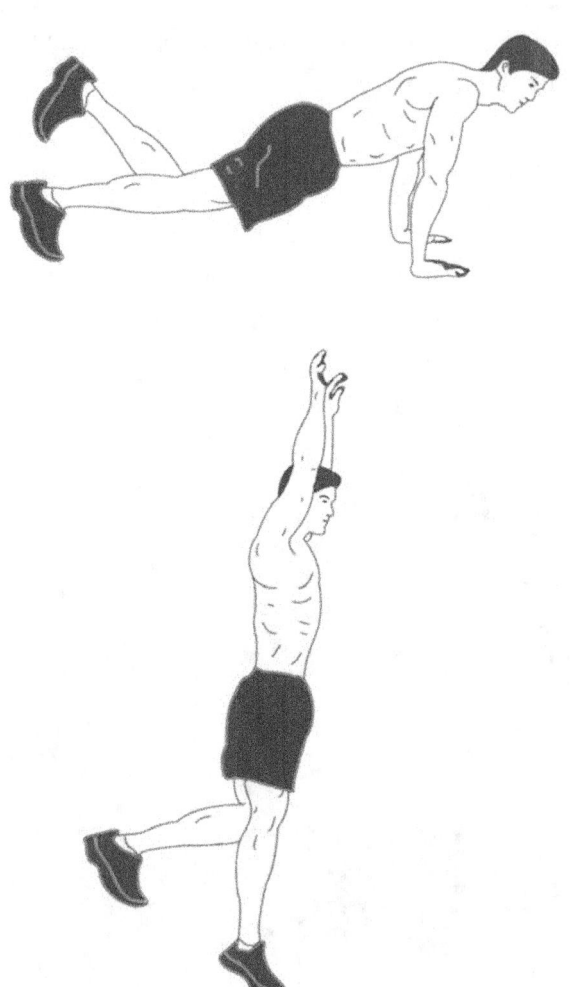

Level 6 Exercise

Pistols

Stand on the ground with your left leg, hover your right foot above
the ground. Place your hands in front of your body, clasped together.
Bend your left knee and lower your bottom to your heel. Keep your
right leg straight and off the ground, as much as you can. Stand back
up with your left leg only. Repeat on the other leg.

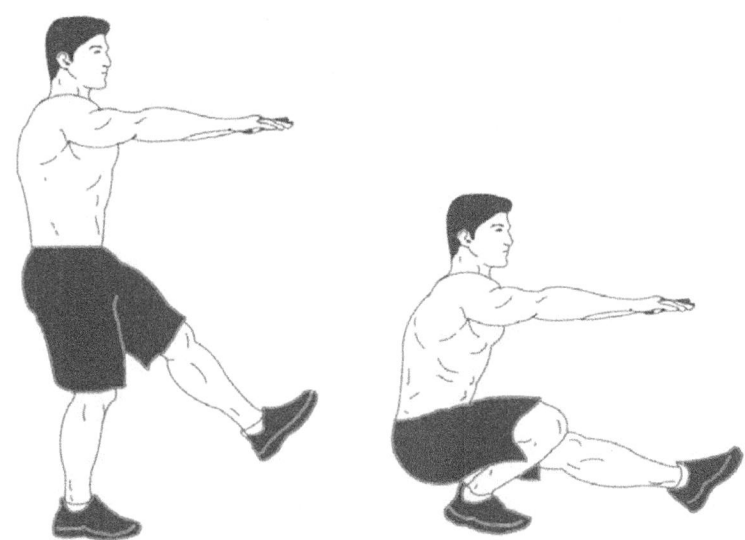

Real High Step (10sec=1rep)

Use a step bench, about 3 to 4 risers underneath. Step up once and return back to original position.

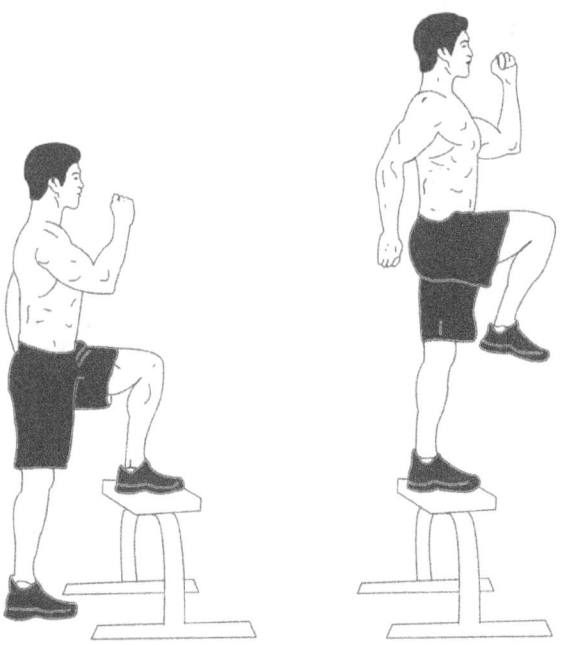

Single Leg Wall Sit (4sec = 1rep)

Stand up with your back against a wall, placing your feet half a foot away from the wall. Your arms should be at your sides. Bend your knees and lower your body until your thighs become parallel to the floor. Form an 'L' with one leg. Hold for 4 seconds. Stay as long as needed and then do the same with the other leg.

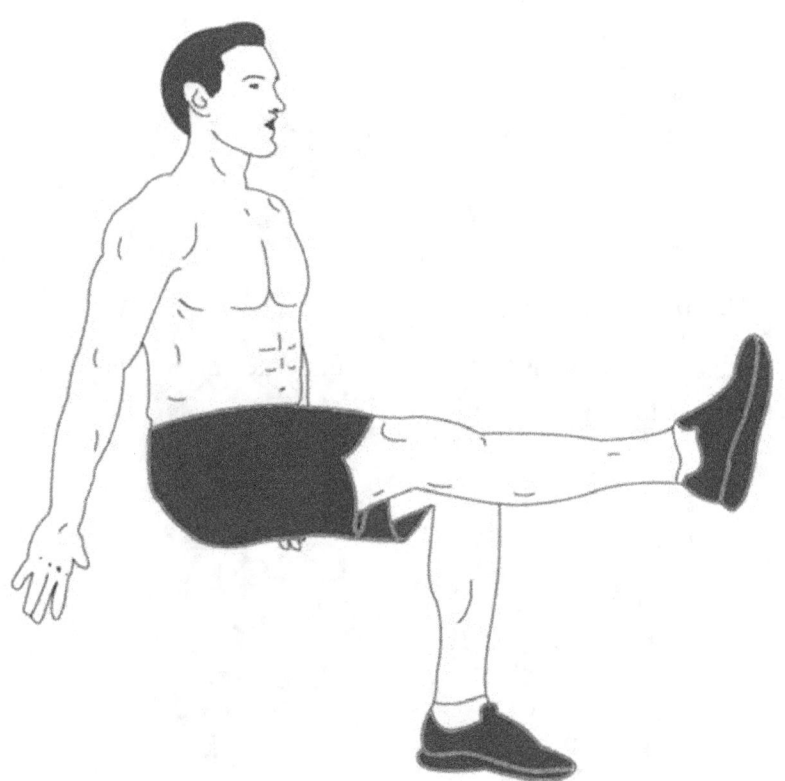

One-Leg Reverse Calf-Raise

Position your heel on the forward edge of a platform. Use your other hand to maintain support. Lift your other leg back by bending your knee. Pull your forefoot up to your body as far as you can and extend your foot until your toes are pointing downward. Switch legs and repeat the steps above.

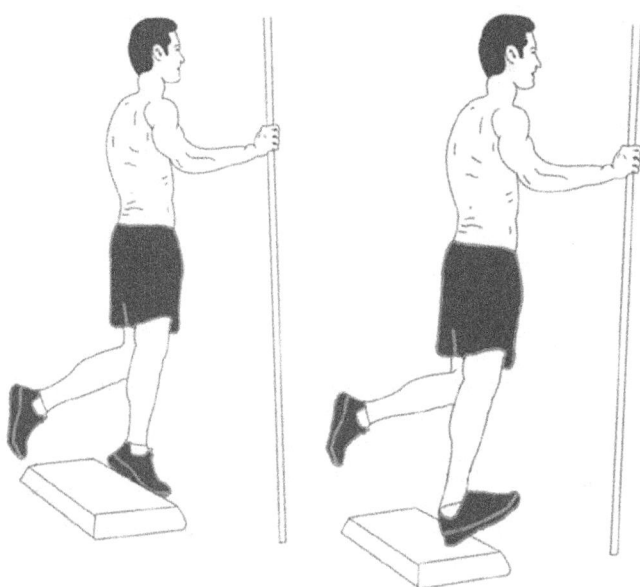

Level 7 Exercise

Do variations of your Leg exercises

For instance: Negative Pistols (8 seconds down, 2 seconds up) (1 negative=4rep)

    Negative Pistols (1negative=2rep)

    Wall sit (10sec=1rep)

Second Bank of Exercises:

Bridge, Flexibility exercises, Yoga poses, Flags and Levers

You can't become a Calisthenics expert without having enough flexibility. This chapter will cover the basics on regular bridge, step-by-step actions on how to properly perform flexibility exercises and yoga poses.

This book wouldn't be a comprehensive and complete guide without a section on how to perform planks, flags and levers.

1. Regular Bridge

For performance purposes, it is recommended you do this 30 minutes prior to training.

Starting Position

Steps to Follow:

Step 1: Lie on your back, with both legs bent and the soles of your feet placed on the floor. Your legs should be adjusted apart to shoulder width.

Step 2: Place your hands above your head and shoulders, palms facing down beside your ears. Your fingers should point towards your shoulders.

Step 3: if you have feeble wrists or wrists that are not flexible, this could be an uncomfortable position. If this is the case, it is recommended you do some regular wrist stretching exercises before you begin the routine, to develop its flexibility.

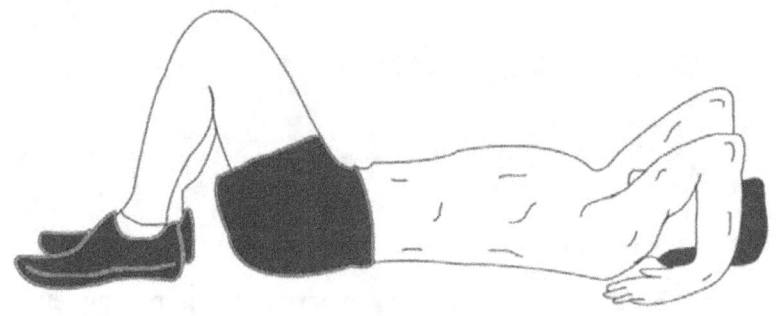

Pushing Up and Collapsing

Steps to Follow:

Step 4: Push your tummy up toward the ceiling, while straightening both arms and legs from the starting position.

Step 5: Bend your back to form an arch and try relaxing in that pose. Hold this pose for 3 - 5 seconds, then slowly and gently collapse back down to starting position.

Step 6: Rest between sets.

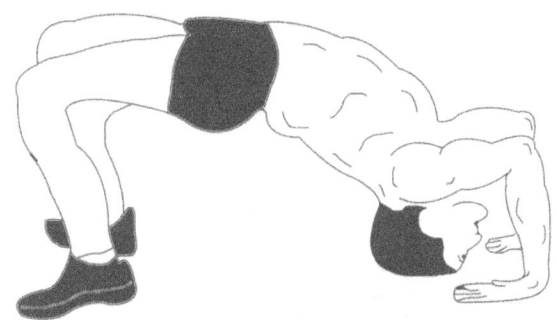

Additional Information

When you rest for a short period, and execute multiple repetitions, you will gain more endurance when doing the bridge faster. This is usual when you put more stress on your muscles, you encourage them to adapt faster.

Please ensure that you don't overdo it to the point of pain. If this happens, stop exercising immediately and rest for a day or more, until you recuperate.

Progressions

You can move on to these progressions once you have built up enough back flexibility and arm strength to hold the bridge for 30 seconds or more.

- Attempt looking up at the sky or ceiling while in the bridge.

- Attempt lifting one foot off the ground and point it toward the ceiling, as high as you can.

- Attempt lifting one foot off the ground and crossing it in a chair position, i.e., the outside of one ankle placed on opposite knee

- Attempt shifting more weight to your arms, by thrusting toward them with your legs. This pose requires that you have more arm flexibility, so do it slowly.

Note: this particular exercise is among several bridge exercises that strengthen your back and avoid back freezes in the future.

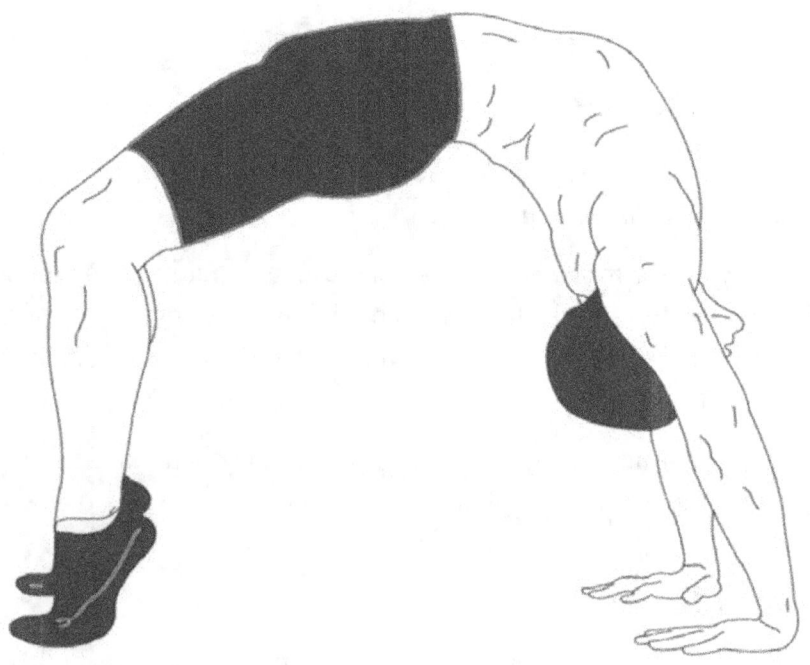

2. Flexibility Exercises

Stretching

Stretching is the most forgotten part of any training and one of the most important. This is an area you don't want to skip at all. Improving your flexibility is a must, if you want to capture the true effects of Calisthenics. Do these stretching exercises after EACH AND EVERY workout, on a mat or on the floor. You can also use some of them for your warm-up.

Precautions

As with any type of workout regime, if you suffer from any medical conditions, it is highly recommended you consult with your physician or a medical practitioner before beginning any training. Medications may need adjusting, diet changed to compensate for the weight loss /muscle gains.

Equipment Required and Other Requirements

- Recommended: exercise mat; but you can use the floor (with some padding)

Hamstring Stretch

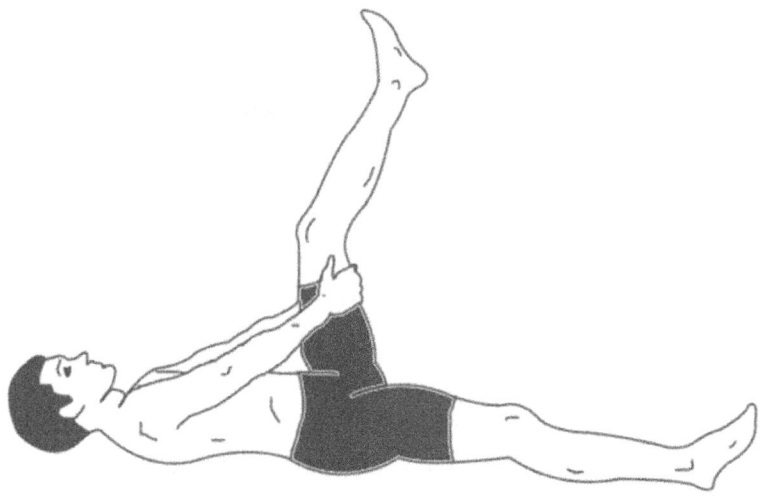

Steps to Follow:

Step 1: Lie on the mat or floor with your knees bent. Lift your right leg off the floor, and hover at your ankle or calf; wherever you can reach.

Step 2: Bend the foot gently, while pulling your leg toward your chest, until you feel the hamstring stretch.

Step 3: Maintain the pose for 15 - 30 seconds. Switch to the other foot and repeat the steps above.

Additional Information

If you feel that your hamstrings are tight or you are generally unstable, use a resistance band to assist you with more leverage.

Hip Flex or Lunge Stretch

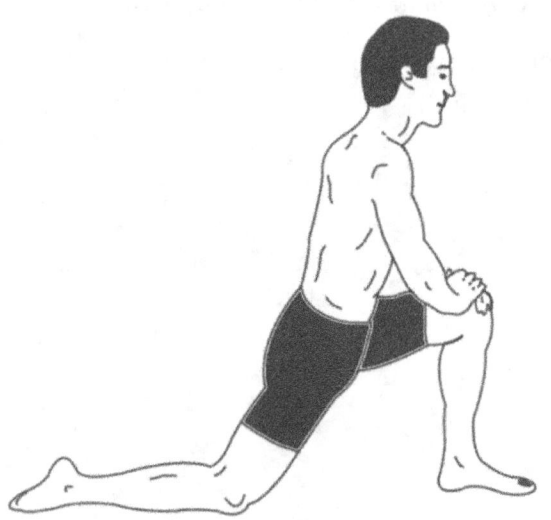

Steps to Follow:

Step 1: Assume a lunge position on the floor, or exercise mat. Place your right foot forward and left knee back. Ensure that both knees form a 90-degree angle.

Step 2: Maintain a straight torso with your abs caged. Lunge forward and gently thrust until you feel the front of your hips extend.

Step 3: Squeeze your glutes for a more profound stretch and maintain this for 15-30 seconds. Switch sides and repeat the steps above.

Kneeling Hamstring Stretch

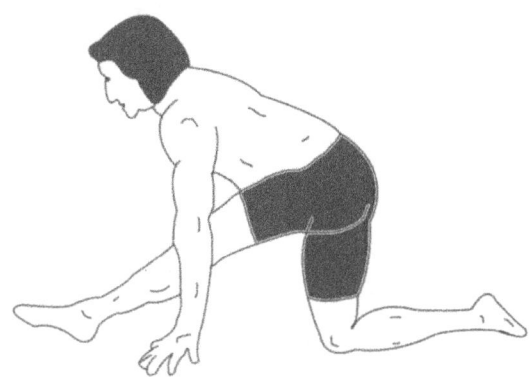

Steps to follow:

Step 1: Assume the normal lunge position. Move back and put your weight on the left knee, while straightening the other leg.

Step 2: Lean forward at the hip, ensuring your back remains flat, until you feel a gentle pull at the back of your leg.

Step 3: Maintain a slight bend in your knee if your hamstrings are stiff, and hold for 15-30 seconds. Switch sides and repeat the steps above.

Pigeon Stretch

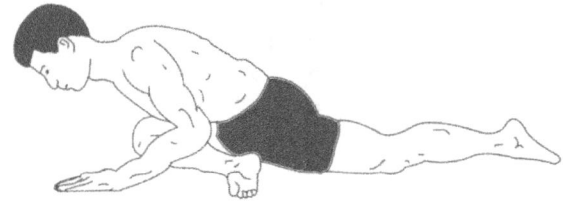

Steps to follow:

Step 1: Begin this exercise on your hands and knees. Bend and slide your left leg in toward your left hand. Press your hips toward the floor.

Step 2: Stretch your right leg out behind your body. Bend forward. Rest your forearms on the floor.

Step 3: Maintain this position 15-30 seconds. Switch legs and repeat the above steps.

Quad Stretch

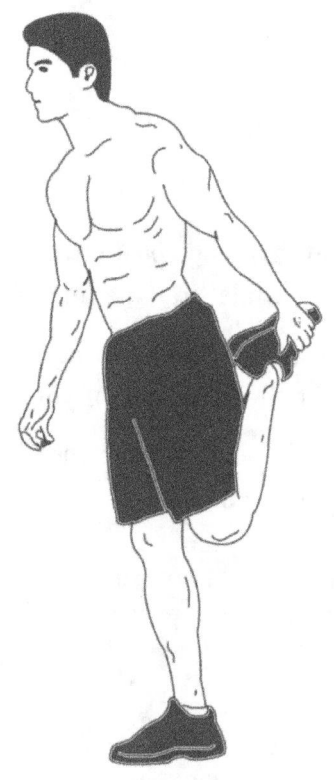

Equipment Required

A chair, bench or a ball

Steps to Follow:

Step 1: Hold onto a wall while standing upright. You don't need to hold the wall if you can maintain body balance.

Step 2: Bend one leg behind your body. Reach back and wrap your hand around the foot of the bent leg. Guide your foot toward your bottom, while ensuring your knee points straight at the floor. If you do this correctly you should feel stiffness right down the front of your leg.

Step 3: For a deeper stretch, you can try to squeeze your hips forward. Maintain the pose for 15 - 30 seconds. Switch sides and repeat the above steps.

Important Information

- Begin with a two to five minute warm up; light cardio or walking

- Maintain each stretching pose for 10-20 seconds.

- If you want to ensure significant results, ensure you do these stretches working out.

- Should you experience any soreness or irritation, cease the exercise until healed.

Yoga Positions

Believe it or not, Yoga positions are by far the best stretching exercises to develop your flexibility.

It is recommended you do these exercises at the end of each training session. It will enhance your flexibility and ability to complete the positions in your workout regime.

Flexibility Exercises with Yoga

Hamstrings

The hamstring muscle is the muscle that runs up along the back of your thigh. These are vital muscles that need to be stretched since tight and lethargic hamstrings usually cause back pain.

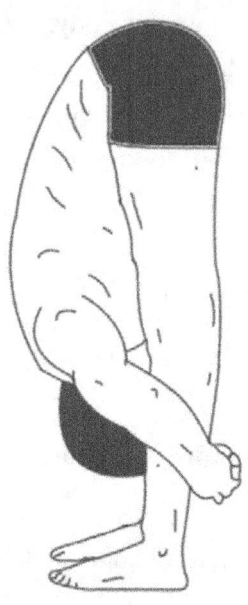

Standing forward Bend – UTTANASANA

The standing forward bend is the easiest way to exercise your hamstrings. Ensure that you place your hips over your ankles; most individuals usually allow their hips to extend too far back.

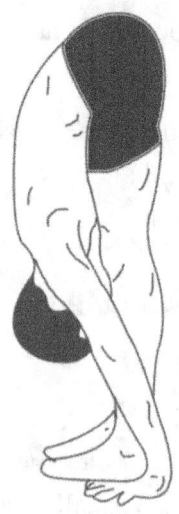

Steps to Follow:

Step 1: From upright stance pose, plunge your arms out to the side, while bending forward.

Step 2: Ensure you are bent from the hips forward and not from the back.

Step 3: Place your fingertips in line with your toes and keep your palms flat.

Step 4: Stretch out the quadriceps muscles of the thighs. Keep in mind that the more you stretch your quads, the more your hamstrings will open up.

Step 5: Thrust your weight further forward, into the sole of your feet, so your hips stay over your ankles.

Step 6: Let your head hover above.

Additional Information

Not everyone is flexible to complete the position. You may need to bend your knees slightly, to keep your palms pressed to the floor. As you become more flexible with each exercise regime, you can attempt to straighten out your legs, while palms pressed to the floor.

Triangle Pose – UTTHITA TRIKONASANA

You will need a yoga block under your bottom hand, especially if you are alone and need help to reach the floor. It is recommended to exert pressure against the block and not your leg. To achieve this effect, you will have to lean on it.

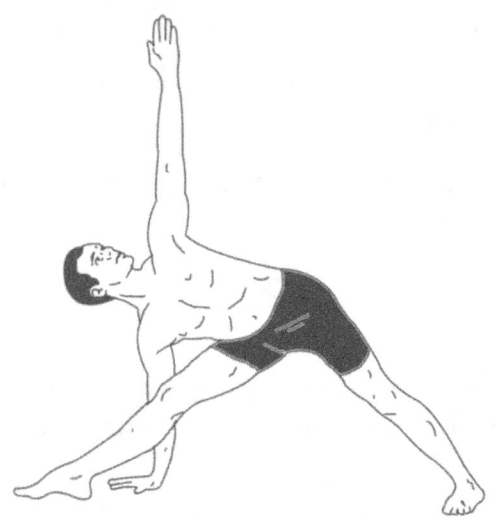

Steps to Follow:

Step 1: From the upright stance, straighten your right front leg.

Step 2: Stretch your right arm out in front of you. Engage your right thigh as you go.

Step 3: Lower your right hand to your ankle or shin. If you are more flexible, lower your right hand to the floor, on either side of your ankle or shin, until you are comfortable.

Step 4: Stretch your left shoulder over to your right shoulder- open your chest. Then stretch your left hand toward the ceiling, extending your fingertips. Make sure your left shoulder stays in place.

Seated Wide-Legged Straddle – *UPAVISTHA KONASANA*

This routine is a good way to stretch the insides of your thighs. The more open you are, will determine how best you can take a forward bend. Try to do it with a straight spine. It could also useful to remain sitting up if you feel that it is more appropriate for you.

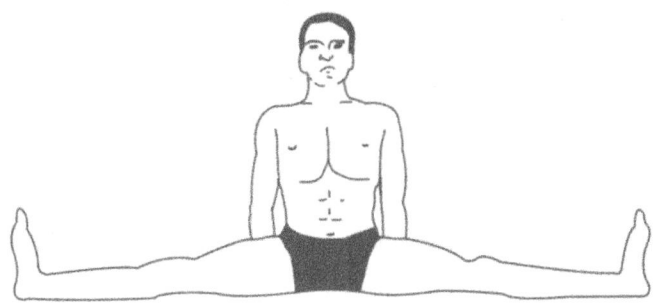

Steps to Follow:

Step 1: From a seated pose, open your legs as wide as you comfortably can.

Step 2: Ensure that you keep your thigh muscles and feet stretched.

Step 3: Ensure that your toes are pointing straight up, to the sky or ceiling.

Step 4: Thrust your legs down into the floor.

Additional information

For beginners, try putting a pad under the buttocks if necessary.

Eye of the Needle - SUCIRANDHRASANA

This is a wonderful pose for individuals with tight hips because it is very diverse.

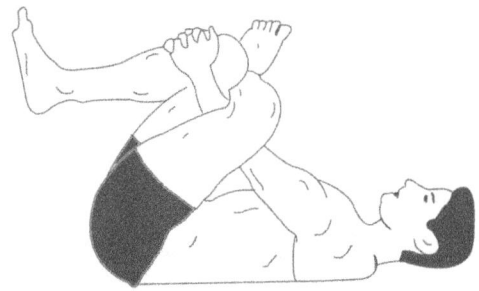

Steps to Follow:

Step 1: Lie on your back with both knees bent. Place soles of your feet against the floor.

Step 2: Lock your left knee into your chest.

Step 3: Crisscross your left ankle over your body, while resting it on the right thigh.

Step 4: Relax your left knee away from your torso.

Step 5: Place both hands on your right shin. Lift your right foot off the floor and thread your left hand through your legs.

Step 6: Use your hands to draw your right thigh toward your chest. This position will open your left hip- feel the stretch.

Step 7: Ensure that both feet are stretched outward.

Step 8: Maintain the relaxed pose- left knee will open your hips. Switch legs and repeat the steps above.

Additional Information

It is recommended that anyone who experiences difficulty stretching or beginners, should not perform the position after step 4, until you have become more limber and practiced the position a few times.

Pigeon - EKA PADA RAJAKAPOTASANA

This routine is an amazing hip opener. However, it can be a vigorous one for people with tight hips. It is recommended you perform the position while using a prop, to maintain your balance.

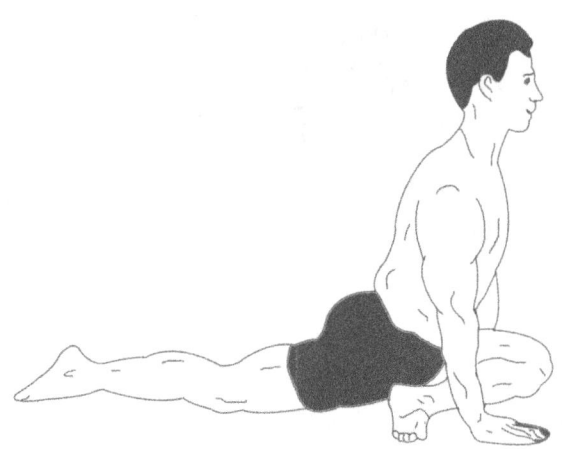

Steps to Follow:

Step 1: With your back bent and hips open, raise your right leg up, into a down dog split.

Step 2: Turn your right knee and bring it to the floor, outside the right hand, as you slide the front of your left leg to the floor. Depending on your flexibility, place the right shin toward your left hip so that it angles back.

Step 3: Place your hips toward the front of the exercise mat or floor.

Step 4: Place the pad under the right side of your bottom. Most people do this in order to make their pose to be more comfortable.

Bridge Pose - SETU BANDHA SARVANGASANA

This exercise offers a proper way to stretch your shoulders, while maintaining the bridge pose. If bending your back is uncomfortable, you can attain a similar stretch in a supported bridge, by performing the same shoulder-tucking process and interlocking your fingers to encompass the block.

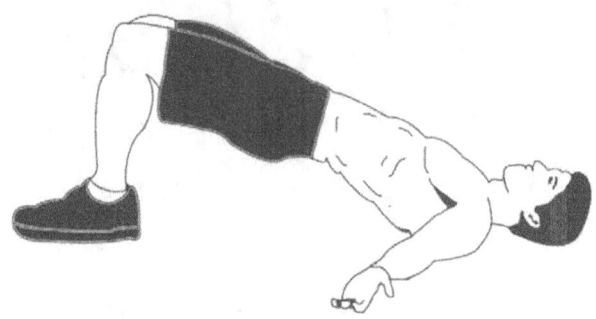

Steps to Follow:

Step 1: Lie on your back.

Step 2: Bend your knees, so the soles of your feet are parallel on the mat and close to your bottom.

Step 3: Lift your hips toward the sky or ceiling.

Step 4: Interlock your fingers behind your back and align your arms, while thrusting them down onto the mat or floor.

Step 5: Spin or twirl one shoulder under, followed by the other arm.

Step 6: Raise the hips higher.

Step 7: Stretch your chest toward your chin- make sure you do not move your chin from your chest.

Step 8: Ensure your feet stay parallel.

Step 9: Release your hands and then bring the upper, middle, and then lower back down respectively.

Step 10: Repose to allow your knees to clip together.

Planks

Planks are a diverse exercise that can be used for many different purposes. In fact, with planks you can replicate many body exercise routines on the ground.

Elbow Plank ("Classic Plank")

This is the most exemplary Plank exercise that you should start with.

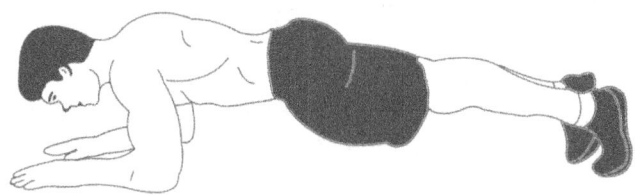

Steps to Follow:

Step 1: Ensure you keep your bottom on the ground, and your head in a neutral pose, i.e., your face is slightly forward. Do not lower your head to look at your toes.

Step 2: Place and maintain your shoulders directly over your elbows, or a little bit forward. However, do not dip behind, as this will drive your bottom up.

Step 3: Clench your bottom and thighs together, to work the muscles. Proceed with the exercise, while breathing normally, and then hold your breath for as long as you can.

Top of Push-Up Plank

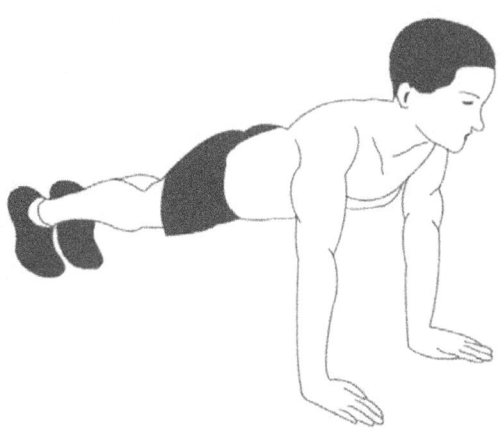

Steps to Follow:

Step 1: Like the Plank mentioned above, stretch your arms outward, as if you are about to perform a Push-Up. Your hands should stay directly under your shoulders.

Step 2: Proceed with the exercise, while breathing normally, and then hold your breath for as long as you can. For so many individuals, this is an easier variation to start with since your body is slightly inclined.

Side Plank

Steps to follow:

Step 1: Rotate your body into the standard Plank. Tuck your elbows under your body.

Step 2: Draw your hips up towards the sky or ceiling.

Step 3: Have your top arm placed either on your hip or have it stretch upwards.

"Tom Cruise" Plank ("Mission Impossible" Style)

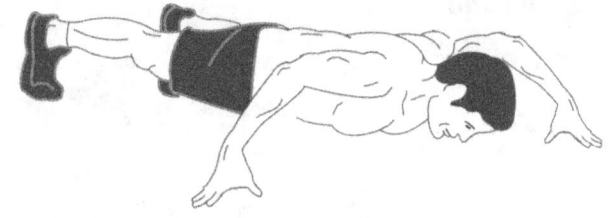

Steps to Follow:

Step 1: Begin the routine in the top of a Push-Up position.

Step 2: Gradually widen your hands and feet as wide as you can manage.

Step 3: Ease your body down toward the ground and hover above the ground.

1-Legged Plank

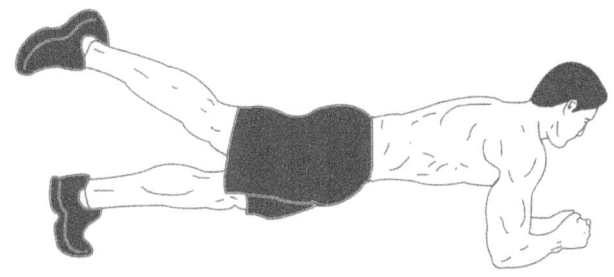

Steps to Follow:

Step 1: Assume the classic Plank position, hen lift one leg off the ground.

Step 2: Maintain this pose for 30 seconds to 2 minutes, then lower your body back to the starting position. Switch to other leg and repeat the steps above.

1-Arm Plank

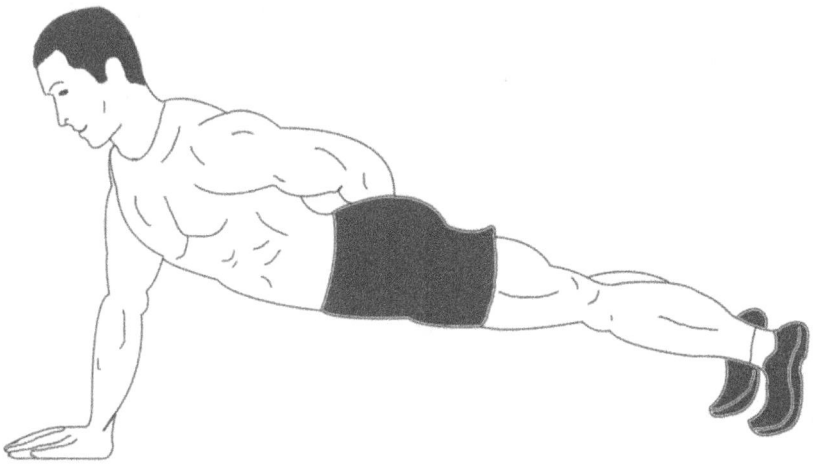

Steps to Follow:

Step 1: Assume the classic Plank position, then lift one arm off the ground.

Step 2: Stretch your arm out away from your shoulder. Maintain this position for 30 seconds to 2 minutes.

Step 3: Lower your body back to the ground. Switch to other arm and repeat the steps above.

Flags

Regular Human Flag

Steps to Follow:

Step 1 (Feet Lifts): You will need a pole to perform this position; but it doesn't need to be a specific type of pole. (The pole can be a dancing pole, street lamp or any other thin vertical object that is stable and you can get your hands around.) Grab the pole firmly with your hands; with your palms facing in the same direction. Bend to the side and attempt to maintain your feet at a level just above the ground. This procedure requires a great amount of body stability and strength. Once you can hold the position, start lifting them jointly until you reach a point where your body is almost parallel to the ground, before you return to the starting position.

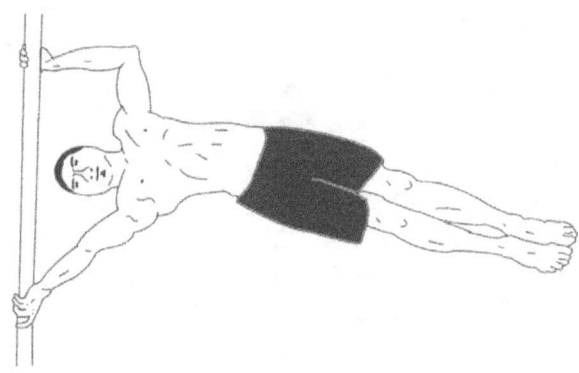

Step 2 (Tuck Flag): The human flag is not an easy exercise; it requires a lot of practice. In this step you will be tucking your feet behind your body, and it will make the position easier to maintain. This will replicate a half-sized human flag.

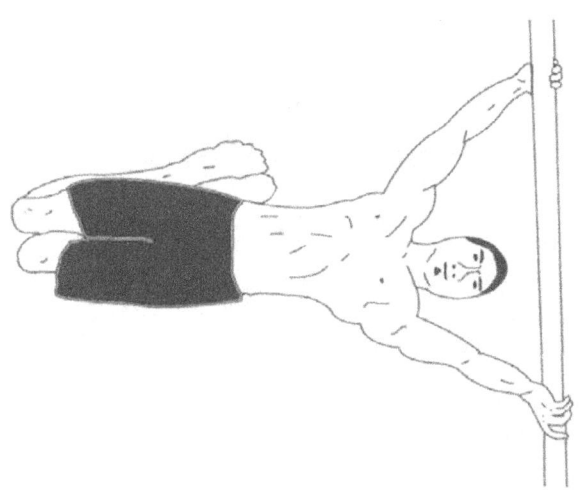

Step 3 (Double Leg Drops): Hold your body up, and beyond the parallel position, which is between 30 to 45 degrees from the ground. Before moving to the starting position, place your legs in parallel position to the ground. This will make it less difficult for you to stimulate full flag. Try doing this exercise by dropping just one leg to the parallel position, and after this you can start using both legs.

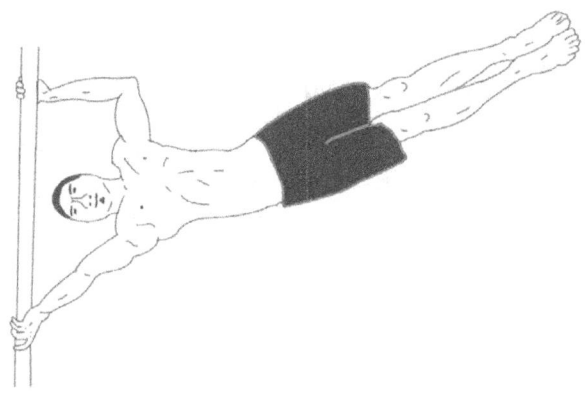

Step 4 (Full Flag): With your body completely parallel to the ground, try to hold the human flag position.

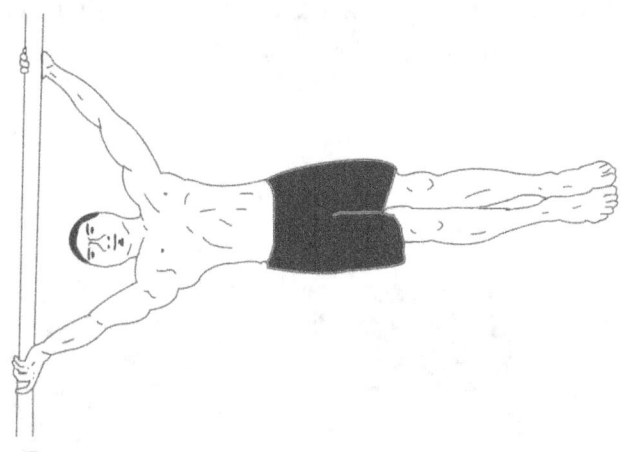

Human Flag Parallel Bars

The human flag is one of the most challenging body weight exercises of all time. In human flag, brute strength is not key to success. For one to achieve a full human flag, you must have a careful and detailed understanding of all the information about it. Be dedicated and patience.

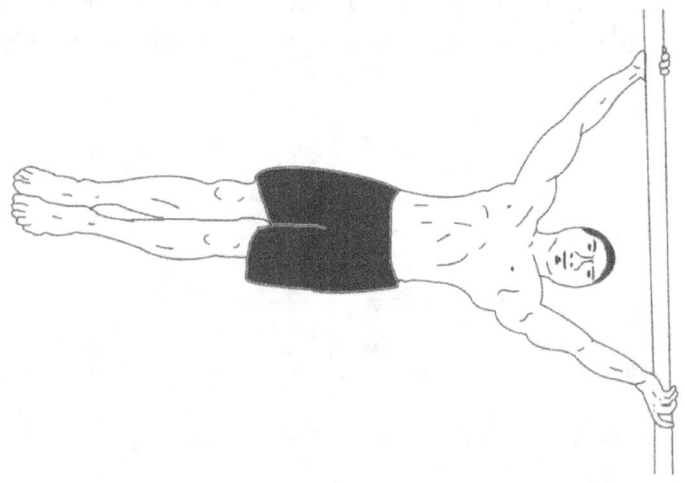

There are two main methods one can perform a human flag; the first one involves both hands grabbing a vertical pole with mixed or overhand grip. The second one is called the human flag on parallel bars and it does not involve use of bars found in dips, but rather bars that are placed vertically in a parallel manner.

Levers

Tuck Negative "Side Lever"

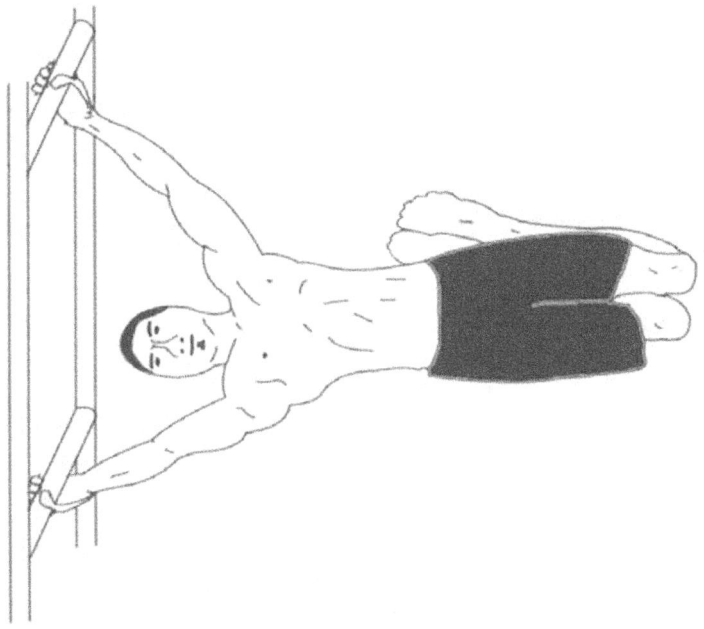

Steps to Follow:

Step 1: Find something you can get your arms around, then get your hands into position and determine your strongest position. Some of the strongest positions include making your palms to face each other, forward or mixed grip. However you decide to place your hands, make sure they are in a straight line which is perpendicular to the ground.

Step 2: After establishing a solid grip, make an attempt of jumping to a completely inverted position and try tucking your legs behind your back.

Step 3: With your legs still tucked behind your back, slowly go all the way down to the starting position, as you come close to the ground make sure your legs don't touch the ground and continue tucking them.

Step 4: Use your strength and stability to go back to the inverted position.

Step 5: Repeat the same procedure several times.

Negative "Side Lever"

You should not attempt this if you are not adequately prepared, or if you are not confident.

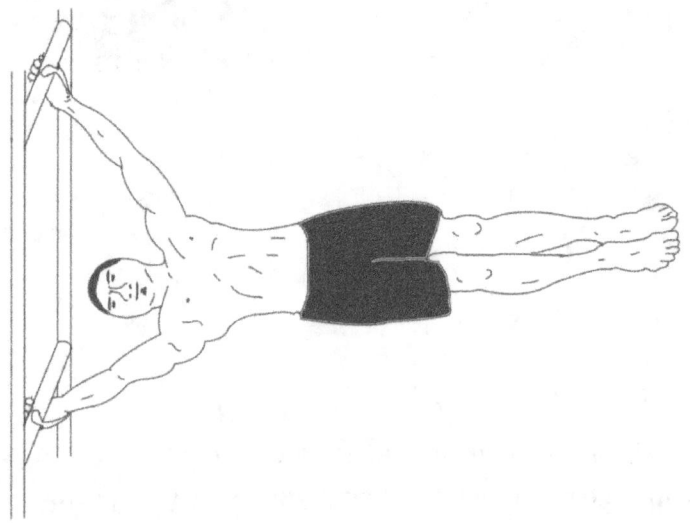

Steps to Follow:

Step 1: Find something you can get your arms around, then get your hands into position and determine your strongest position.

Step 2: After establishing a solid grip make an attempt to jump into a completely inverted position- making sure your legs are straight. For you to achieve this, you should ensure the firm pressure with your bottom arm is maintained. You should also note at the inverted position, your body will no longer be fully sideways.

Step 3: With your legs straight, slowly go all the way down to the starting position. As you come close to the ground, bend your legs (tuck them behind your back) so they don't touch the ground.

Step 4: Use your strength and stability to return to an inverted position.

Front Lever Raises/Pulls

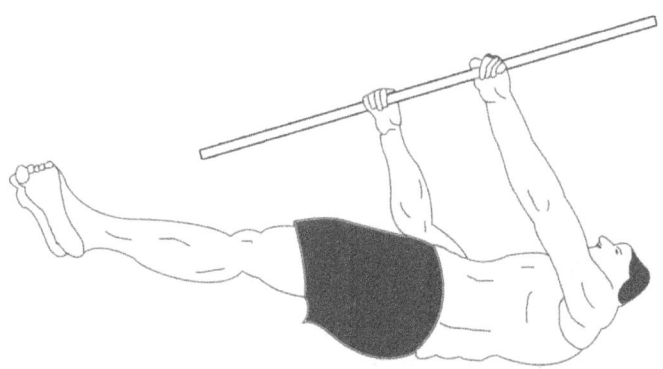

Grip the bar with palms facing away from your body. Keep your body straight, with your hands a bit wider than shoulder width. Pull yourself a bit up and lean back. Bring your feet up in the air, making your body parallel to the ground. Hold this position for 2-4 seconds, slowly lower your feet back down.

Flag Pulls

Flag pull is considered to be an advanced movement. For you to perform it, you have to be comfortable with being a static human flag, and make sure you execute the pose correctly. After having mastered it, you can take a step higher on your progressive Calisthenics journey to perform flag pulls.

Flag Pulls (Upper Half)

https://www.youtube.com/watch?v=x0Lsp_6V47E

From: 6:24 to 6:32

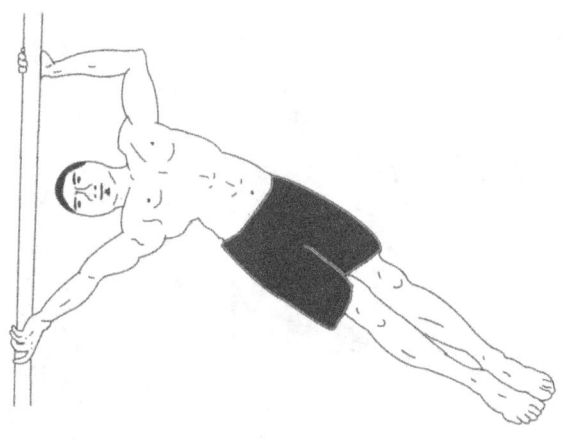

Steps to Follow:

Step 1: Find something you can get your arms around, then get your hands into position and determine your strongest position.

Step 2: After establishing a solid grip, make an attempt of jumping to a completely inverted position, making sure your legs are straight. For you to achieve this, you should ensure the firm pressure with your bottom arm is maintained.

Step 3: With your legs straight, slowly go all the way down, to mid-point or until your body is perfectly horizontal.

Step 4: Use your strength and stability to return to inverted position.

Flag Pulls (Lower Half)

https://www.youtube.com/watch?v=x0Lsp_6V47E

From: 6:32 to 6:38

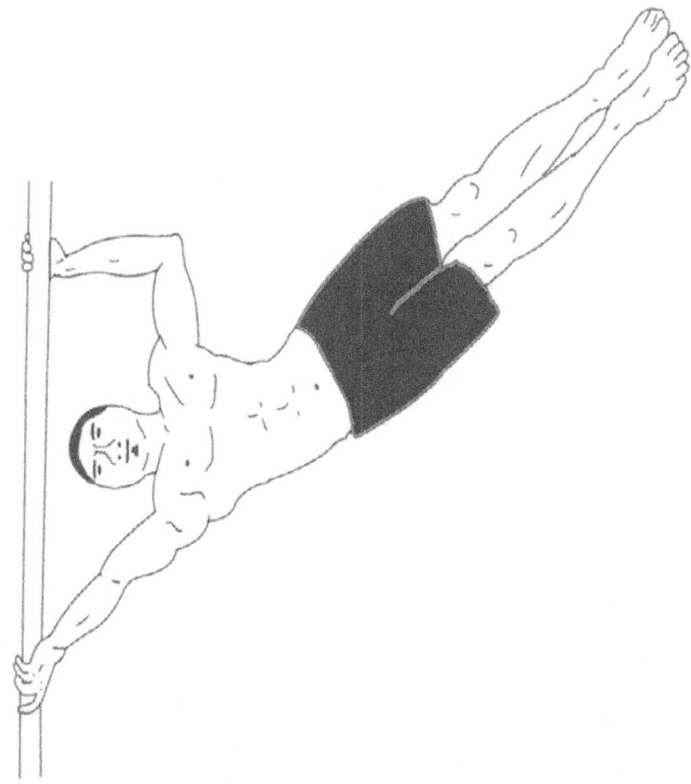

Steps to Follow:

Step 1: Find something you can get your arms around, then get your hands into position and determine your strongest position.

Step 2: After establishing a solid grip, try jumping to a mid-point or until you reach a perfectly horizontal position, make sure your legs are straight. For you to achieve this, you should ensure firm pressure with your bottom arm is maintained.

Step 3: With your legs straight, slowly go all the way down to the ground, but don't let your legs touch the ground. Keep your legs straight throughout the exercise.

Step 4: Use your strength and stability to mid-point or perfectly horizontal position.

Full Flag Pulls

https://www.youtube.com/watch?v=x0Lsp_6V47E

From 6:40 to 6:45

Steps to Follow:

Step 1: Find something you can get your arms around, then get your hands into position and determine your strongest position.

Step 2: After establishing a solid grip, try jumping to a completely inverted position, making sure your legs are straight. For you to achieve this, you should ensure the firm pressure with your bottom arm is maintained.

Step 3: With your legs straight, slowly go all the way down to the ground, but don't let your legs touch the ground.

Step 4: Use your strength and stability to return to inverted position.

Section 5:
YOUR DIET

By following this program, you will experience ultimate strength and muscle gains. But without a good diet, you won't have the best gains you could have.

If you are ready to follow the Calisthenics diet and want to maximize your workout efforts, commit yourself to eating right and declare war on junk food. Self-discipline is a must and strictly following limited calorie intake will help you achieve your dream body. Once you are determined about eating healthy, the rest is easy.

There are so many ways to eat healthy. The volume of calories we consume regulates body weight. Everything you do burns calories, including sleeping, digesting food and even breathing. Actually, any addition to what you normally do, burns calories. Therefore, diet and exercise should be collaborative! That's why they are commonly found in sentences, together.

There are many people determined to lose weight and eliminate fat from their bodies. They also realize it is a gradual process, like most things in life. It takes time and plenty of effort to achieve a healthy body and fit form. No good results came from rushing the process. There are actually rules to follow in a diet, especially when you are in a Calisthenics program.

5 Rules You Must Follow

Eat real and natural fats

Do you think that eliminating fat will help your diet? We actually need certain fats in our body. In fact, it is an important part of a healthy diet; they provide fatty acids, keep our skin soft, produce fat soluble vitamins and are a great source of energizing fuel.

Basically, there are two types of fats; the good and the bad. Both of these, when consumed in moderation, can be used to replace saturated fats or bad fats, Good fats can mostly be found in vegetable oils. An example of good fat, is Omega-3, which can be found in fatty fish (salmon, catfish, mackerel), as well as flaxseed and walnuts. Fats that can be found in fruits are the monounsaturated fats, which are typically liquid at room temperature, but it turns solid when refrigerated. They can be found in avocados, olives, almonds, hazelnuts, cashews, sesame seeds, canola and peanut oils.

Bad fats have two types; saturated and trans-fat acids, both of these fats can raise cholesterol levels, increase heart disease and clog arteries. Saturated fats are commonly found in animal products; such as, meat, poultry skin, high-fat dairy, and eggs. They are also available in vegetables; that are liquid at room temperature; such as, coconut and palm oil. Fat is everywhere and all we can do is be aware of what we eat, and exercise.

Here are some tips to help you reduce the amount of fat in your diet, and to make sure the fats you consume are the healthy ones.

- Try a vegetarian meal, with plenty of beans, once a week
- Select dairy products that are skim, or low-fat
- Choose a diet rich in whole grains, fruits, and vegetables.
- Replace fattier sauces with vinegar, lemon juice, and mustards.
- Try using olive oils instead of plain palm oil or coconut oil

Those are a few things you can practice to minimize your fat intake, the most important thing is awareness and knowledge about fats, and self-motivation to avoid them.

Avoid Sugar and Processed Carbs

What is the difference between a sandwich made on white bread and one made on 100% whole grain? The difference between French fries and a side salad made with spinach, tomatoes, carrots and kidney beans? All of them are carbohydrates.

It is not about totally avoiding sugar, it is simply lowering your intake, to reduce the risk of diabetes and maintain a balance in your body. We need sugar in order to survive, you just need to control the amount and how you get it.

When it comes to carbohydrates, it can also be good or bad. It is how we get it and the amount consumed. We can benefit from good carbs, by choosing carbohydrates full of fiber. These carbs get absorbed slowly in our systems, reducing the spike in blood sugar levels. We can also minimize the health risk of bad carbs, by eating fewer refined and processed carbohydrates that strip away the beneficial fiber. For example, white bread and white rice, both high in carbohydrates.

Too much of anything is not good for your body. Moderation is key to maintaining a healthy lifestyle. And exercising is good for your body too!

- Make sure to eat a balanced diet, with sufficient calorie intake, helps in building muscle. If you need additional calories, 200-300 will do, no more.

You will learn the importance of strictly following rules and setting up goals. If you want to achieve a muscular body, you need to love yourself and implement self-discipline as well. Your diet includes eating 1 apple a day, and you have been following it for weeks, then 1 day you forget, now that's a big change because your body adapted to the vitamins the apple gave, is interrupted by missing 1 day of eating it.

Every human being has a number, of Basal Metabolic Requirement; the amount of energy in the form of food calories (kcal's) that one requires to do nothing but lay in bed and not move, the bottom line, bare minimum one must have to maintain cellular function.

The root here is the importance of nutrition, whether you are a bodybuilder, athlete or a calisthenics master, your nutrition is the most important component, next to training, not only for gaining quality muscle but also to achieving lean body mass, gains, and strength. There is an approach of eating everything in sight. This approach is when you eat everything and anything, all for the sake of calories.

Ask yourself, would you eat a high-carb meal just before sleeping, when carbohydrates are your body's main source of energy. Sounds like a very tricky question but it's not. A simple logic that really makes sense. With regards to calories, why would you take more than suggested daily calorie intake, when you can be strong enough with that amount? Calisthenics is about self-discipline and inner strength- a physical strength resulting in a very healthy life, in body and in mind.

Eat 4 Times Per Day. No More, No Less

With obesity becoming one of the most common problem around the world, you may have heard about the importance of eating in small portions. Right? No matter if you are concerned about your weight, your energy level or nutritional deficiencies, eating small portions can help maintain optimal health. There are some very important things we need to consider, and remember to answer the question, why do we have to eat 4 times a day or in small portions.

First, when you eat less, you decrease your daily calorie intake

One of the most important reasons that you should eat small portions is in doing so, you are decreasing your chances of developing obesity. It doesn't matter how many or what size of meals you eat, but rather a total amount of food you eat each day.

Maintains Blood Sugar Levels

Eating small amounts helps maintain a constant blood sugar levels. Blood sugar in a human body helps to give you energy throughout the day. Therefore, a low blood sugar level makes you feel tired, slow and sluggish. Each time a person eats, the body releases blood sugar from the food. If you eat small meals frequently, you will receive a steady stream of blood sugar, thereby preventing blood sugar crashes. In contrast, if you eat larger portions only one or twice a day, your blood sugar will spike much higher after eating these meals, and similarly will crash a short while later. This is very dangerous for people with diabetes or are insulin dependent.

Prevent Metabolism Crash

Maintaining an even metabolism is a very important function of the body, as it works to digest food. By eating more often, you are boosting your metabolism and, therefore, will keep it working constantly to digest and reduce the fat in your body, among other benefits. In contrast, when you eat large amounts at each meal, at a more frequent rate, your metabolism experiences lags when it is not active. Eventually, your metabolism begins to slow the pace at which it works. This can result in rapid weight gain, and later, on to obesity.

Prevent Nutrition Imbalances

Eating small portions, several times per day, will help to prevent nutritional imbalances. Research has found that people who eat several different meals throughout the day, tend to eat a different thing at each meal; thereby getting a balanced diet of fruits and vegetables, lean meats, and fiber. A Nutritional imbalance is a factor that will affect your diet. You may think that you are physically fit because you are thin but inside you, there is an imbalance which later on will show its effect.

Eat Protein and Fat Every Meal

Regardless of the past success with fat-restricted diets, lowering fat intakes doesn't equate with dropping fat. A little fat in your diet can be beneficial. Studies made by scientists about muscle building and fitness, have revealed that the right amount of protein and fat every day, in every meal, does help. Not only in fat burning but in regulating blood flow. When you look at the macronutrient percentage of your diet, everything needs to add up to 100 percent. Everything needs to be balanced, that's why it's called balanced diet.

Eating more carbs means eating less fat, and vice versa. From a fat loss perspective, displacing carbohydrates by increasing fat in your diet sets the stage for an optimal fat loss environment. Eating fat every day also enhances your body's ability to burn fat, which is a big help in muscle building.

For meals- be sure to include both protein and a healthy fat, and remember you can mix and match items within a category, as long as the total proportion makes sense. A tuna salad for your lunch, you could use 2 tablespoons of chopped olive (full serving would be ¼ cup) and 2 tablespoons safflower mayo (2 -4 tablespoon for full serving), or you could use 2 tablespoons of olive oil for a salad dressing, and add a handful of sliced almonds to your salad. This is a good example of balance protein-fat diet.

3 Principles

1. You should know how many calories you must eat per day. There are a bunch of websites where you determine your level of calorie intake.

2. Know how many proteins your body needs to build muscle.

    Lean Mass Weight (Kg) x 2.75= Daily Protein Requirement

3. Record everything. I personally use the app called MyFitnessPal. *As Greg Plitt said, "Record everything; what you eat, your training habits, and how you feel."*

Carb Cycling Diet

Carbohydrates are used as energy by the body, they fuel workouts. As well as providing ample fuel to be used throughout the course of the day. Ingesting carbs also replenishes our glucose and glycogen stores, to prevent fatigue.

Carb-cycling allows you to still eat carbs, from clean sources, without adding body fat, and cycling enables you to better utilize fat for burning. It is a method of making use of good carbs for your benefit. Carbs is not a bad thing, if incorporated with a diet properly.

Repeating this cycle throughout the diet plan will boost your system, and allow your body to adapt. There are also examples of clean carbs you can use throughout your diet, such as potatoes, Yams, Brown Rice, Oatmeal, Cream of Wheat and Grits.

Carb-cycling is considered to be the most effective diet to build muscle. In my book "Carb-Cycling: Everything You Need To Know About Carb-Cycling (Bonus And Recipes Included)," I explain step-by-step the JOCCAE (John O'Malley Carb Cycling Anabolic Environment), which is a carb-cycling type of diet.

Bonus Section: Delicious Recipes

BREAKFAST: LOW CARB

OMELET WITH SALMON AND ASPARAGUS

4 oz salmon, diced

½ tsp cooking oil

2 Tbsp onion, diced

1 clove garlic, chopped

2 asparagus spears, diced

¼ tsp lemon juice

2 eggs

1 tsp low-fat milk

¼ tsp dill, chopped

½ Tbsp parsley

Dash of salt

Dash of pepper

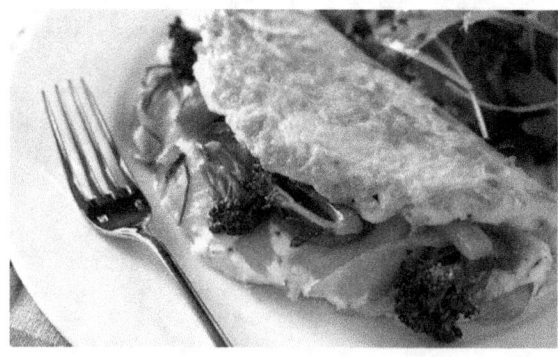

Directions:

1) Rinse the asparagus. Break off the wooden ends. Chop the asparagus into bite-size pieces.

2) In a medium-sized pan, heat the oil. Add the onions and asparagus, allow them to sweat, approx. 2 minutes.

Add the chopped garlic and lemon juice. Cook for 2 minutes.

3) In a separate bowl, mix the eggs. Add the milk, parsley and salt and pepper. Pour into the pan with other ingredients.

4) Add the salmon and allow the eggs to cook. Transfer to a plate. Top with the chopped dill. Serve hot. Enjoy!

MEDITERRANEAN OATMEAL

½ cup oatmeal

1 cup vegetable stock

1 tsp dried oregano

1 Tbsp olive oil

1 clove garlic, diced

¼ cup kalamata olives, chopped

¼ cup dry tomatoes, chopped

¼ cup feta cheese, crumbled

Dash of pepper

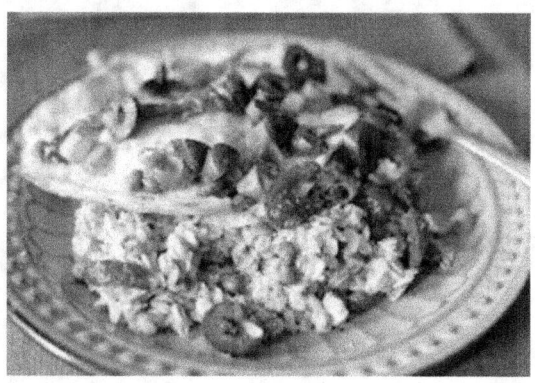

Directions:

1) In a medium-sized pot, combine the vegetable stock, oregano, oatmeal, pepper. Bring to a boil, reduce the heat. Cook for 5 minutes.

2) In a separate pan, heat half of the olive oil. Cook the garlic and tomatoes until tender

3) Once the oatmeal has absorbed most of the vegetable stock, take the pot off the heat and cover for 2 - 3 minutes.

4) Pour into a bowl, top with the cooked vegetables, chopped olives and crumbled feta cheese. Drizzle the rest of the olive oil over the top. Serve hot. Enjoy!

Lunch:
MOZZARELLA AND TOMATO SALAD

1 medium tomato, cubed

1 oz mozzarella cheese, cubed

1 cup spinach leaves

1 clove garlic, chopped

1½ tsp olive oil

2 Tbsp balsamic vinegar

2 tsp sunflower seeds

¼ tsp black pepper

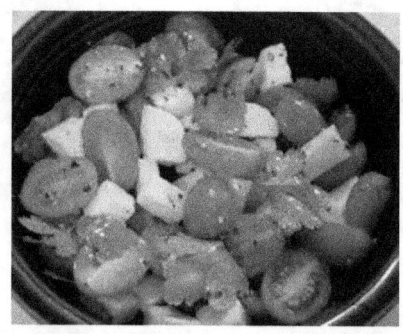

Directions:

1) In a medium-sized serving bowl, add the chopped vegetables.

2) Add the liquid (olive oil, balsamic vinegar). Add the sunflower seeds, pepper. Mix everything together. Serve cold. Enjoy!

AUTUMN PUMPKIN MIX

¾ cup Brussels sprouts

1 cup pumpkin, cubed

1 Tbsp olive oil

1 oz goat cheese

2 Tbsp pistachios

½ medium pear, sliced

2 Tbsp balsamic vinegar

2 tsp yellow mustard

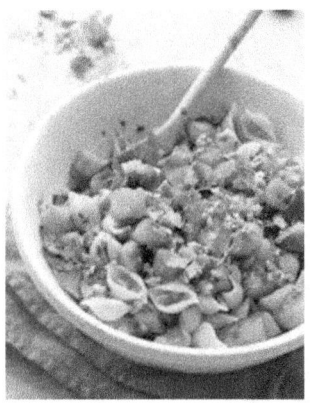

Directions:

1) In a medium-sized sauce pan, heat half of the olive oil. Cook the cubed pumpkin and Brussel sprouts, until they are softened.

2) As they cook, in a small bowl, add the other half of olive oil, balsamic vinegar, and yellow mustard. Combine thoroughly.

3) Once the vegetables are softened, add the sliced pears. Heat thoroughly.

4) Pour the cooked veggies and pears into a serving bowl, add the liquid dressing. Mix until everything is coated. Top with pistachios and goat cheese. Serve warm. Enjoy!

Dinner:
MEDITERRANEAN LENTIL SALAD

2 cups water

½ cup dry lentils

1 can chickpeas, drained and rinsed

½ yellow bell pepper, sliced

1 red bell pepper, sliced

1 carrot, grated

1 cup lemon juice

2 Tbsp olive oil

½ cup fresh cilantro, chopped

Dash of salt

Dash of pepper

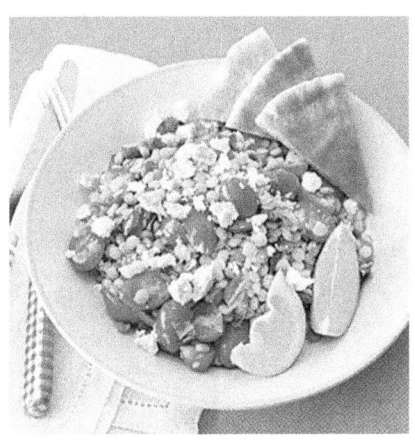

Directions

1) In a medium-sized pot, heat the water until boiling. Add the lentils, cook until tender. Drain the lentils.

2) In a medium-sized pan, heat half the olive oil. Add the cooked lentils, bell peppers, carrots, tomatoes, chickpeas. Cook until they are softened.

3) Add the lemon juice. Combine and heat thoroughly.

4) Pour into a serving dish. Drizzle the remaining olive oil over the ingredients. Top with fresh cilantro, salt and pepper. Serve warm. Enjoy!

SMOKED MACKEREL SANDWICH

1 large garlic

8-10 Tbsp extra
virgin olive oil

Nine ½ thick, slices
Italian bread

Bunch of small
arugula leaves

3 smoked mackerel

fillets ($^3/_4$ lb)

(Skinned, broken
into chunks)

½ red onion, thinly sliced

1 medium tomato,
thinly sliced

Dash of salt

Dash of pepper

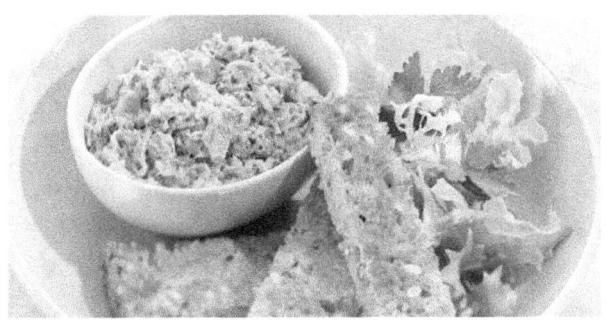

Directions:

Preheat oven to 350F

1) Slice off the top of the garlic bulb, Drizzle 2 - 3 Tbsp olive
oil over the open bulb, rub it in gently with your fingers.

Wrap the garlic bulb in aluminum foil- wrap it loosely, and firmly close all the edges. Bake 40 minutes and set aside (leave it wrapped).

2) Place the slices of Italian bread on a cookie sheet, drizzle olive oil over each piece. Grill the bread until lightly toasted. Remove from the oven.

3) In a small bowl, extract the roasted garlic, mash it up with a fork. Add 2 - 3 Tbsp olive oil, salt and pepper. Mix well.

4) Now, build your sandwich. Lay the grilled bread on a plate. Spread the garlic mixture evenly over the slices of bread, then layer the arugula leaves, onion slices, tomato slices. Top with chunks of mackerel. Serve and Enjoy!

Dessert:

DIPPED STRAWBERRIES

1 ½ sweetened, shredded coconut; toasted

¾ finely chopped salty peanuts or chocolate sprinkles

¾ cup strawberry jam

24 large strawberries, washed

(Leave stems on strawberries)

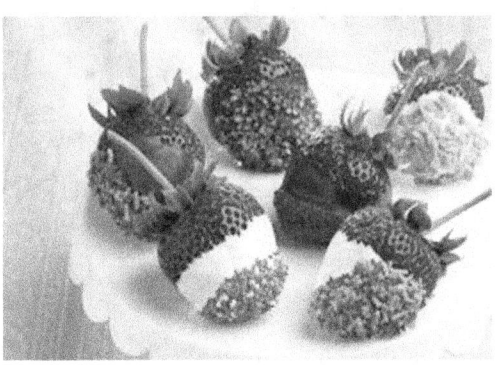

Directions:

1) Dip a strawberry in the jam, then dip in chopped peanuts or sprinkles. Place on a tray. Pop them in the fridge. Chill for 1 – 2 hours. Serve cold. Enjoy!

CARAMELIZED PLUMS

1 Tbsp water

1 Tbsp unsalted butter

$^1/3$ cup granulated sugar

1 pinch kosher salt

5 Plums, cut into wedges

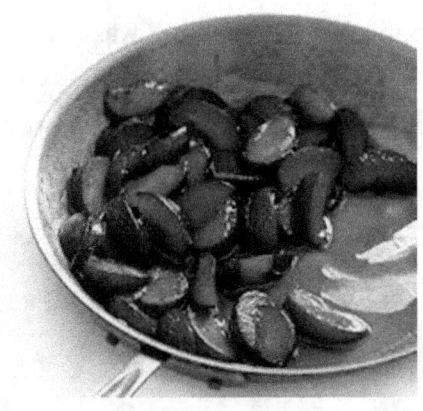

Directions:

1) In a medium saucepan, melt the butter. Add the sugar, salt and water. Mix. Heat until the liquid becomes thick.

2) Once the mixture is a thick consistency. Add the plums. Stir to evenly coat the plums. Simmer for 3 minutes. Serve warm. Enjoy!

Breakfast:
HIGH−CARB DAY

Spicy Grilled Pork and Grapes Kebabs

1 ½ tsp curry powder

¼ tsp cumin

¼ tsp paprika

2 Tbsp olive oil

3 Tbsp orange juice

Garlic, finely chopped

1 lb pork tenderloin, bite-size cubes

¼ pound large, firm seedless grapes

1 – 2 Tbsp parsley, coarsely chopped

Dash of coarse salt

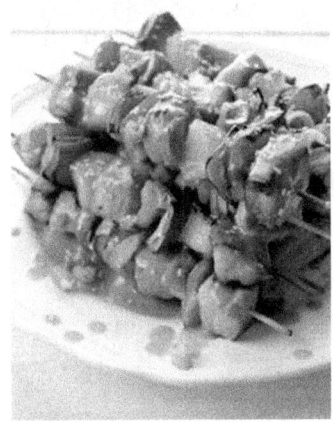

Directions:

1) In a small bowl, combine the curry powder, cumin, paprika and cinnamon. Cover with plastic, set aside.

2) In a large bowl (deep enough to dip a skewer), combine the orange juice, olive oil and garlic. Mix well.

3) Thread the pork and grapes on skewers- depending on the size of the meat and grapes, you should get about 3 -4 of each per skewer.

   Now this is where you decide between two methods for marinating your skewers.

4) You can rub the seasoning onto the skewered meat and grapes, then pour the liquid over the skewers.

   OR

5) Dip the skewers in the liquid, place them in a single layer, in a deep dish and sprinkle the seasoning over the skewers, turning them once during the seasoning.

6) Whichever route you choose, after seasoning the skewers, pour the rest of the liquid into the pan with the skewers, cover with plastic and place them in the fridge to marinate, for 1 hour to 1 day. Rotate the skewers halfway through marinating.

7) Heat your grill to medium-high heat. Place the skewers on the grill and reduce to medium heat. Depending on the size of your pork, Cook the skewers for 8-12 minutes. Turn once.

8) Place the skewers on a serving dish. Sprinkle with parsley and coarse salt. Serve hot. Enjoy!

Lunch

PASTA WITH FETA CHEESE AND TOMATOES

1 package linguine

¾ cup dried tomatoes

¼ cup basil leaves

2 Tbsp almonds

2 Tbsp parmesan cheese

1 Tbsp garlic, minced

½ tsp salt

¼ tsp black pepper

½ cup feta cheese, crumbled

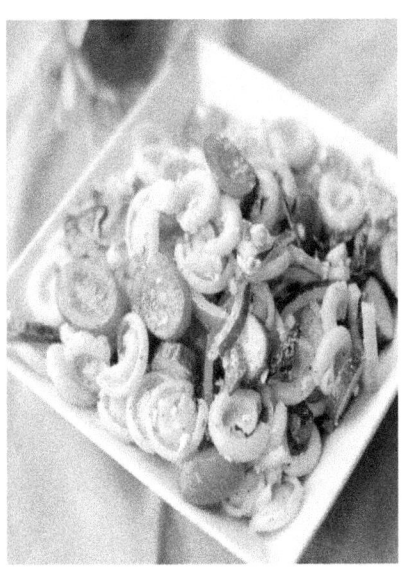

Directions:

1) In a large pot, cook the linguine according to package directions.

2) While the pasta cooks. In a food processor, add the tomatoes, basil leaves, almonds, parmesan cheese, garlic, salt and pepper. Pulse until thoroughly combined.

3) Set aside ½ cup of the pasta water. Drain the linguine. Pour back into pot. Add the mixture from the food processor. Add a bit of the pasta water and stir. (If it still seems dry, add a bit more of the water, stir.)

4) Pour into a serving dish. Top with crumbled feta cheese. Serve warm. Enjoy!

Dinner:

CHICKEN CORDON BLEU

2 pcs boneless, skinless chicken breasts

2 slices ham

4 slices swiss or cheddar cheese

4 Tbsp bread crumbs

2 Tbsp Flour, to coat chicken

1 large egg

Pinch of salt

Dash of black pepper

Glass Baking dish

Optional: ¼ tsp paprika

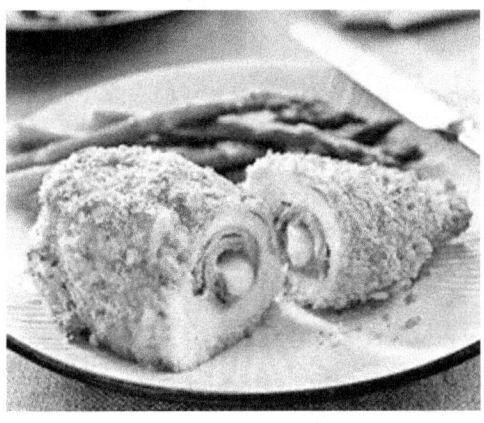

Directions:

Preheat oven to 375F

1) Rinse the chicken breasts in cold water, pat dry.

2) Place a chicken breast between 2 pieces of waxed paper or in a Ziploc baggie. Using a rolling pin or mallet, pound the chicken breast to ¼ inch thickness.

3) Place the coating mixtures into separate bowls. Flour (+optional paprika) Egg, slightly beaten Bread Crumbs

4) Preheat the oven. As it preheats, slip the glass baking dish into the oven. (This keeps the dish hot so when you add the browned chicken breasts, it continues to cook.)

Now, let's roll your chicken breasts, and get them oven-ready.

5) As you begin to roll your chicken with the other ingredients. On the stovetop, heat a medium-sized skillet to high heat, coat the bottom of the pan with olive oil.

6) On a plate, lay the chicken breast flat, place 1 piece of ham and 2 pieces of cheese (but not all the way to the edge, so it doesn't ooze out).

7) Dip the chicken breast in flour, coat both sides.

8) Dip in the egg, coat both sides.

9) Dip in bread crumbs, coat both sides.

10) Place the coated chicken breasts into the heated skillet. Brown on both sides. Pop them into the preheated glass baking dish. Cook for 30 – 45 minutes.

11) When you take the cooked chicken out of the oven, let it sit for 2 minutes. Using a sharp knife, slice the fillets into ½ inch slices. Serve hot. Enjoy!

Q. & A. SECTION

What are the requirements? What can I do to maximize the effectiveness of the training?

A great diet is a must if you want results. I can't recommend enough you get my book titled, "Carb-Cycling: Everything You Need To Know About Carb Cycling," a results-oriented diet book where I explain in detail the JOCCAE (John O'Malley Carb Cycling Anabolic Environment). Consume your daily protein requirement and follow the advice I gave you in the diet section included in this book.

Daily protein requirement: 2.75 x Lean Muscle in kg

Lean Muscle: Weight - (Weight x BF)

As for any supplements, you can take 5g of creatine monohydrate right after training, with 40g of whey protein. I don't recommend any other supplements.

Another important component to successful training, is sleep. This training is super-intense, so you need to make sure you have enough rest. Sleep more than usual, and at least 7h30 per night.

I'm already an expert who can do the 3 sets/14reps of the hardest exercises. What can I do?

I recommend you perform even harder exercises; add heavier weights.

Should I cycle this training?

Yes you should. As I told you at the very beginning of the training, you will complete 3-day routine for 6 weeks, then take a week off, in which you can do some cardio, improve your flexibility, and learn new movements. Still, stay at 50% of your maximum potential. Then, do the 4-day routine for 6 weeks. Repeat.

Can I do Calisthenics 2.0 for years? Is there any risks that I stop progressing?

There isn't. Moreover, you should do Calisthenics 2.0 for years because always changing routines won't improve your strength and muscle mass. Why? Well, basically your nervous system "learn and register" how to perform a movement, and "register" the order of the exercises of a specific training. Always changing requires your nervous system to continuously adapt and "learn," which prevents your muscle from focusing on performance. Learning new exercises is enough. Don't waste too much time on changing routines every other week, just because you think it will "shock your muscles." A muscle doesn't get shocked. It's a muscle.

Arms are my weakness. I can't progress enough and it prevents me from performing a lot of exercises. My arms aren't big enough. What can I do?

I've created a program called, "7-Day Arm-Blasting To Gain Up To An Inch In 7 Days," because a lot of people I know are facing, or have faced this exact issue. This program isn't for weak people. It's hard. If you are just looking for a 1-month pump just to "beef" up, this isn't for you. If you are really serious about getting bigger arms in a ridiculous amount of time, I recommend the Arm-Blasting program. You will experience massive, unprecedented life-time gains.

Chest is my weakness. I can't progress enough and it prevents me from performing a lot of exercises. / My chest isn't big enough. What can I do?

Same thing here. I created a program called, "7-Day Chest-Blasting To Gain Up To 3 Inches In 7 Days," for the same reasons. People have had the same extraordinary results, because the program is based on the exact same principles as in the Arm-Blasting program.

How can I contact you?

I would love to hear from you. If you have any question, or you want to share your results. You can write me: johnomalley.calisthenics@gmail.com

All my books are available on Amazon. I invite you to check them out!

CHECK OUT MY OTHER BOOKS

1) Diet books

The ultimate diet to lose weight, gain muscle mass and be lean:

Carb Cycling – Everything You Need To Know About Carb Cycling (30+ Recipes And Bonus Included):

Honestly. My other 2 diet books are really great but if you had to pick only one book to improve your health and physical strength, pick the one above.

Ketogenic Diet: Everything You Need To Know About The Ketogenic Diet (40+ Recipes And Bonus Included):

Atkins diet: Everything You Need To Know About The Atkins Diet (40+ Recipes And Bonus Included):

2) Bodyweight training books

Calisthenics: 7-Day Arm-Blasting Calisthenics Workout To Gain Up To An Inch In 7 Days:

Calisthenics: 7-Day Chest-Blasting Calisthenics Workout To Gain Up To 3 Inches In 7 Days:

All my books are available on Amazon. I invite you to check them out!

CONCLUSION

I hope you enjoy this program and I hope you are working hard on it. You can continue this program as long as you want, you will keep growing, becoming stronger and healthier, while having the body that you deserve.

I really hope you appreciate my work. If so, could you please leave a comment on Amazon? I would love to know how it works for you. It is why I do what I do. I want to inspire people to take action, and provide them with the best information I can Calisthenics is a lifestyle, and Calisthenics 2.0 is the guide.

The next step is to continue to grow. To work harder. To perform each, and every day, at your best. The last step is to inspire others, so they can take charge of their lives too!

Let's Get Fit Calisthenics 2.0 lovers,

John O'Malley

www.ingramcontent.com/pod-product-compliance
Lightning Source LLC
Chamberburg PA
CBHW071358280526
45787CB00001B/371